KNOWLEDGE MEANS EMPOWERMENT.
TEST YOURSELF.

1. What is the leading natural cause of death among women?
2. What simple exercises can help stop stress incontinence—and make sex more pleasurable?
3. What can cause vertigo in women in their 50s?
4. What medications can cause constipation in older women?
5. What is a frequent cause of ulcers in older women?
6. What percentage of arthritis sufferers are women?

ISN'T IT IMPORTANT THAT YOU HAVE THE FACTS? YOUR LIFE AND YOUR HEALTH MAY DEPEND ON THEM.

Answers:

1. *Cardiovascular disease*
2. *Kegel exercises*
3. *Ménière's disease*
4. *Calcium channel blockers, calcium supplements, aluminum-containing antacids, narcotics, and some antidepressants*
5. *Aspirin and aspirin-like medication, such as ibuprofen*
6. *70 percent!*

Books by the American Medical Women's Association

THE WOMEN'S COMPLETE HEALTHBOOK
THE AMWA GUIDE TO NUTRITION AND WELLNESS
THE AMWA GUIDE TO PREGNANCY AND CHILDBIRTH
THE AMWA GUIDE TO FERTILITY AND GENETICS
THE AMWA GUIDE TO EMOTIONAL HEALTH
THE AMWA GUIDE TO SEXUALITY
THE AMWA GUIDE TO CANCER AND PAIN MANAGEMENT
THE AMWA GUIDE TO AGING AND WELLNESS
THE AMWA GUIDE TO EARS, NOSE, AND THROAT
THE AMWA GUIDE TO CARDIOVASCULAR HEALTH
THE AMWA GUIDE TO INTERNAL DISORDERS

The American Medical Women's Association

Guide to Aging and Wellness

Medical Co-editors
Roselyn Payne Epps, M.D., M.P.H., M.A., F.A.A.P.
Susan Cobb Stewart, M.D., F.A.C.P.

A Dell Book

Published by
Dell Publishing
a division of
Bantam Doubleday Dell Publishing Group, Inc.
1540 Broadway
New York, New York 10036

This material was originally published along with other material in *The Women's Complete Healthbook* published by Delacorte Press.

Illustrations by Wendy Frost

ISBN: 0-440-22307-5

Reprinted by arrangement with Delacorte Press

Printed in the United States of America

Published simultaneously in Canada

December 1996

10 9 8 7 6 5 4 3 2 1

The AMWA Guide to Aging and Wellness

Roselyn Payne Epps, M.D., M.P.H., M.A. and
Susan Cobb Stewart, M.D. Co-editors

Whether monitoring personal health care or caring for aging family members, women need a definitive resource for accurate, dependable, and up-to-date information. *The AMWA Guide to Aging and Wellness* presents the essential components of overall good health for women fifty years of age and older, as researched by the American Medical Women's Association (AMWA), the most historic and prestigious association of women physicians in the United States. Knowledge of physical, mental, and social concerns is crucial for detecting the early signs of many illnesses and for preventing potential diseases. Women must be prepared to handle some of the changes and concerns that affect them as they grow older.

AMWA believes that women must avoid a disease-oriented approach to women's health and focus on maintaining optimal health on a daily and long-term basis. The more one knows about one's body and its functions, the better equipped one will be to safeguard good health into advancing years through preventive strategies such as eating properly and exercising regularly. The content of *The AMWA Guide to Aging and Wellness* is organized into four major sections, each of which stresses the importance of preventive medicine and encourages total body awareness to avoid health problems that specifically affect aging women.

Part I, Aging, describes the biological process of growing older. It alerts the reader to the many changes that occur in women's bodies as they age—such as urinary incontinence and calcium deficiency—and advises how to maintain good health with regular exercise, proper nutrition, regular screening tests, and a healthy lifestyle. This section also includes specific information on older women's medication options, such as hormone replacements and painkillers.

Part I also discusses menopause, informing the reader about this natural but nevertheless difficult phase of every woman's life. It provides useful information about the symptoms, physiological changes, emotional impact, and medical implications of menopause. Since hormone therapy has become commonplace in handling many of the side effects of menopause, this section discusses a range of hormone treatments, such as estrogen and progestin supplements used to control osteoporosis and cardiovascular disease. The changes in sexual activity, which are common as a result of altered hormone levels later in life, are also addressed in this section.

Part II, The Brain and Nervous System, presents a plan for maintaining health and alertness for women concerned with their aging mental faculties. Although preventive care and diagnostic tests can reduce the chances of developing nervous system disorders, it is still important for women to know how the brain and related neurological systems function. Strokes and memory loss are potential problems, but regular visits to a physician and avoiding substances such as tobacco and alcohol are some commonsense steps that women can take to avoid them.

Part III, The Musculoskeletal System, educates women on how the muscles and bone structures work, and provides advice for maintaining full range of motion and comfort into older age. Arthritis, the most common inflammatory joint disease, affects almost 30 million American women; osteoporosis, resulting from bone loss, is another potentially dangerous condition affecting women over 50. This section outlines the major musculoskeletal disorders and treatments, in areas ranging from back, hip, foot, and joint pain to electromyography, arthroscopic surgery, and joint replacement procedures—and specifically relates these issues to the aging female body.

Part IV, Cancer in Women, alerts women to the risks and symptoms of cancer development. Cancer occurs more frequently among people over the age of 65, at which point it becomes a serious health issue. As with many disorders, being familiar with the risk factors of cancer—from genetics and environmental factors to diet, sunlight, and tobacco use—can prompt aging women to seek medical attention and potentially speed up the process of early professional diagnosis. Although each woman's case requires individual health care for treating cancer, a general discussion of the various methods available—including radiation, surgery, and chemotherapy—will make women over 50 aware of their options.

The AMWA Guide to Aging and Wellness provides authoritative information that aging women need to prepare themselves for growing older in today's changing environment. It illuminates the health concerns unique to mature women of the 1990s and offers sound medical advice. Supported by the expertise and experience of the American Medical Women's Association, *The AMWA Guide to Aging and Wellness* is a comprehensive approach to health maintenance and wellness for women who would like to look forward to health and fulfillment in their golden years.

CONTENTS

The American Medical Women's Association

Guide to Aging and Wellness

PART I

Aging

Judith C. Ahronheim, M.D., F.A.C.P.

The population of the United States is aging rapidly. By the year 2030, nearly 22 percent of the population will be over the age of 65 years. Average life expectancy has been increasing steadily since the turn of the century. To a large extent this is due to the decrease in the death rate of infants. The average life expectancy of a woman is 7 years longer than that of a man. It is estimated that a woman who lives to age 65 can expect to live an additional 19 years.

The gain in years lived at midlife and beyond can be a mixed blessing. Chronic diseases occur more often in the elderly, and the years gained may not necessarily be ones of good health and function. There is some evidence that women can expect to live a smaller portion of their lives free of disability than men.

A healthy lifestyle, preventive care, and increased awareness of the special health needs of elderly women can help improve the quality of their lives. Many conditions that affect older women can be prevented or relieved through lifestyle modification and early medical care.

THE DEMOGRAPHICS OF AGING

As women age, they confront some difficult social issues. In comparison to men, older women are more likely to be unmarried, to live alone or in an institution, and to rely on others for support, both financial and otherwise.

Because women live longer than men, the ratio of women to men increases with age. This difference is most pronounced after the age of 85, when there are approximately two and one-half times more women than men. As a result, more women than men live alone for longer periods. The differences in living arrangements are related not only to the longer life span of women but also to the fact that men tend to marry younger women and that divorced or widowed men are more likely than women to remarry.

Among those living in an institution, the ratio of single (widowed, divorced, or never married) women to men is much higher than it is among the elderly who do not live in institutions. Approximately 90 percent of the oldest residents of nursing homes are women. An older woman is more likely to live in an institution if she has survived her spouse or her spouse is too sick to take care of her.

Caregivers of elderly people tend to be women. Of those who provide care to elders in their activities of daily living, 72 percent are women, mostly wives and daughters. These caregivers spend an average of 4 hours a day assisting their elders. Those employed outside the home frequently need to curtail their paid work time to perform these functions. Many spend far more than 4 hours a day in these activities, and some must rearrange work schedules or leave their work altogether.

Some older people who depend on the care of others are subjected to abuse by their caregivers. Such abuse is not necessarily active but may result from neglect.

The financial status of older women is substantially below that of older men. In 1992, the median income of older women was only 56 percent of that of older men. Approximately 16 percent of women 65 and older, compared with 9 percent of men the same age, live below the poverty level. The highest poverty rate is among elderly African-Americans, followed by Latinos. It is estimated that 63 percent of African-American women 75 years of age and older are poor.

In contrast to racial differences in economic status, older African-American women may be healthier than white women. Although average life expectancy at age 65 is approximately equal for African-American and white women, at older ages African-American women can expect to live 1 or 2 years longer. Education improves this advantage. An 85-year-old African-American woman with more than 12 years of formal education can expect to live 3.6 years longer than her white counterpart.

Increasing age increases the risk of disability and the need for assistance in the activities of daily living, such as shopping, cleaning, grooming, cooking, bathing, and going to the bathroom. Among people age 65 and older, approximately 1 in 16 require such assistance, and as a person ages that figure increases to 1 in 2 by age 85. Chronic illness, such as arthritis, hearing impairment, visual impairment, and heart disease are common. Although these diseases do not necessarily impair function, they do increase the risk of disability. The disability rate seems to be declining slightly in recent years, however, and the decline is more pronounced among women than men. This may be related to improvements in recognizing and correcting disabilities, as well as increased use of devices that allow disabled people to be more independent.

THE BIOLOGY OF AGING

It is hard to define a normal aging process. Each person ages uniquely, depending on genetics, lifestyle, and exposure to agents in the environment. Because the prevalence of disease is high in later life, it can be difficult to distinguish a normal aging process from a disease process.

Some people view aging as a buildup of disease. Therefore death can be avoided only if disease could be completely eliminated. The control of some infectious diseases has prolonged survival into midlife and later, when survivors are more vulnerable to diseases of later life, such as cancer and atherosclerosis, a buildup of plaque that causes arteries to narrow and leads to strokes and heart attacks. As certain diseases are eliminated, however, new ones emerge.

The total absence of disease is more a theory than a reality. When certain human cells are allowed to grow in a laboratory, they divide only a finite number of times, and then the normal process of cell multiplication stops. This pattern of "pure aging" (senescence) has been seen in many species, although the precise number of cell divisions varies. It has been suggested that a biologic mechanism, a sort of programming built into cells before birth, determines life span. This program, in addition to other factors, may determine how long humans and members of other species live.

Some scientists believe that factors in the environment affect the aging process. Free radicals have been linked to aging; these excited molecules react readily with many substances including tissues in the body. Humans are constantly exposed to free radicals from the environment; they are by-products of most functions of the body as well. There is evidence that free radicals have a part in diseases such as arteriosclerosis (thickening of the walls of the arteries leading to heart attacks and strokes), cataracts, and cancer. Free radicals may damage the makeup of cells, causing the aging process to speed up. It is difficult to distinguish free radical damage leading to the degenerative diseases of aging from the pure process of aging. Although evidence suggests that free radicals damage cells in tissues, there is little evidence that this promotes senescence.

Certain enzymes, or antioxidants, produced by the body reduce the damage caused by free radicals. Other antioxidants include beta carotene (a member of the vitamin A family), vitamin E, and vitamin C. Current research focuses on how these and other components may affect heart disease, cancer, and visual disorders. Since women have been underrepresented in studies of antioxidants and heart disease, the effect of these and other nutrients remains unclear.

A great deal of attention has been devoted to research on antioxidants and other dietary modifications and their effect on the degenerative diseases of aging and longevity. The effectiveness of these or other strategies is controversial. Proving whether a certain approach prevents cancer is difficult because cancer can take up to several decades to develop. There also is evidence that deficiencies in antioxidants cause certain diseases.

It is premature to recommend specific strategies to prolong women's life span. However, lifestyle modifications, such as healthy diet, smoking cessation, regular exercise, and early cancer detection can help prevent premature death from disease in most people.

A HEALTHY LIFESTYLE

As women live out their later years, they must be able to enjoy their later years to the fullest extent. One way to do this is to lead a lifestyle that promotes health, lowers risks, and in general helps them feel better. Routine health care allows disorders to be detected in their early stages, when they are more easily treated. A healthy diet and exercise program can help prevent some health problems in older women and improve how they look and feel. Preventive health care and some simple adjustments in lifestyle can go a long way in improving women's quality of life.

Routine Care

Many older women do not regularly see a doctor, even though they had routine examinations when they were in their reproductive years. The risk of disease as a person ages makes it imperative that women over age 65 see their doctors for exams and screening tests on a regular basis.

During a routine visit the doctor performs a physical exam that includes a pelvic exam, and checks your blood pressure, height, and weight. The doctor or nurse should ask you about your general health status as well as other aspects of your mental and physical condition that could affect your health. On the basis of this discussion, certain tests are recommended and, if necessary, treatment and follow-up visits are planned.

Screening tests are done when a person isn't sick. They are often done in a general population to detect disease, and sometimes are done if a disease isn't present but the risk is higher. Mammography is very important for older women because the risk of breast cancer rises with age. Other screening tests are recommended at regular intervals as a woman ages. Certain tests are recommended for all women over 65 (see "Routine Care for Women 65 Years and Older"). Additional tests may be suggested based on a woman's history ("Additional Evaluations Based on Risk Factors").

Diet, Nutrition, and Weight

Elderly people can have special nutritional requirements. It may be necessary for a woman to alter daily dietary intake based on her nutritional status, medical disorders, and the drugs she takes. In general, American women should strive to maintain a low-fat diet to lower the risk of cardiovascular disease and stroke and to include adequate amounts of calcium and fiber to meet their changing health needs. However, these rules do not apply to everyone.

Calcium can help prevent bone loss caused by a condition called osteoporosis in older women. How much calcium you should take and for how long is still unclear. Even so, the National Institutes of Health has recommended that postmenopausal women consume 1,500 milligrams per day of calcium. Foods rich in calcium include dairy products, fish, spinach, and vegetable greens. For example, there are 302 milligrams of calcium in one 8 ounce cup of skim milk. Supplementation may be needed, but excess calcium intake should be avoided. Consult your physician about the type and amount of calcium to take (see Part III).

Older women often complain of constipation. A diet high in fiber (the portion of plant food that the body eliminates without digesting) improves gastrointestinal function and may help to control weight and cholesterol if it replaces a high-fat diet. Foods rich in fiber include fruits, vegetables, and grains.

People often gain weight as they age. Their metabolism becomes slower and they need less food to maintain the same weight. Although modest weight gain is not thought to be harmful at older ages, being overweight (20 percent or more than usual or optimal weight) can pose health risks for women with high blood pressure and diabetes. An exercise program, combined with a healthy diet, can help burn off more calories as well as prevent problems linked to being overweight. Unplanned weight loss late in life is usually a sign of a serious problem. Weight loss also can occur in people unable to obtain food, such as those with memory loss, physical disabilities, or limited financial resources.

Loss of appetite is not a part of normal aging, but there may be a delay in recognizing and managing nutritional deficiencies in older people. Many nutritional deficiencies that occur in older woman are related to their poor health. Feeding disorders may be temporary. For example, frail patients may stop eating when they are ill but gradually their appetites return as they gain strength.

Patients may stop eating or need to be fed at a very slow rate at frequent times throughout the day; to satisfy their nutritional needs, tube feeding is sometimes suggested. Fluids and nutrients, or pureed foods, are supplied through a tube inserted into the stomach via the nasal passages or through the wall of the abdomen. Patients have the right to refuse tube feeding, either on their own, through written instructions like a living will, or through someone designated to act for them, just as they have the right to refuse any other form of medical treatment.

Hormone Replacement Therapy

On average, at around age 51 or 52 a woman goes through menopause, although for many women it occurs a decade earlier or several years later. At the time of menopause, a woman's ovaries stop producing the hormone estrogen and she stops having menstrual periods. When this occurs, certain changes take place in a woman's body. She may experience hot flashes, night sweats, or difficulty sleeping. While these symptoms are temporary, other changes are taking place that have more long-term, less obvious effects. They include osteoporosis, bone loss that occurs with reduced estrogen levels, and cardiovascular disease. A lack of estrogen also can cause dryness of the vagina, which is noticeable during sex, as well as increase the risk of bladder infections and urinary tract problems.

To prevent these changes and the problems they

ROUTINE CARE FOR WOMEN 65 YEARS AND OLDER

Screening Tests	Interval
	(may vary—ask physician)
Pap test to detect cervical cancer	Yearly
Blood glucose test for diabetes	Yearly
Mammography for breast cancer	Yearly
Total cholesterol and HDL cholesterol	Consult physician but at least once
Fecal test for occult blood to check for silent bleeding in digestive tract	Yearly
Flexible sigmoidoscopy to examine the colon and rectum for signs of cancer	Every 3–5 years
Thyroid-stimulating hormone test to check for thyroid disease	Every 3–5 years
Hemoglobin and ferritin level to check for iron deficiency	Consult physician but at least once

Immunizations

Tetanus-diphtheria booster	Every 10 years
Influenza vaccine	Yearly
Pneumococcal vaccine	Once

can pose, therapy can replace the estrogen no longer produced in the body. However, although estrogen may be highly effective in suppressing hot flashes, its use for other conditions is less certain, particularly late in life. Because giving estrogen alone increases the risk of cancer of the lining of the uterus, it is given with another hormone, progestin, which protects against this cancer. The protective effect of progestin may make the estrogen less effective in preventing cardiovascular disease, but

ADDITIONAL EVALUATIONS BASED ON RISK FACTORS

Evaluation	Who Is at Risk
Urinalysis for protein	Women with diabetes
Skin exam	All women, especially those often exposed to sun, with fair complexions, or previous skin cancer
Tuberculosis skin test	Women in close contact with someone who has TB; medically underserved, low-income populations; residents of long-term-care facilities
Lipid profile	Women with coronary heart disease
Colonoscopy	Women who have bowel or colon disease or a family history of colorectal cancer
Fecal test for occult bleeding and hemoglobin and ferritin tests	Women regularly taking aspirin or NSAIDs for arthritis
Glaucoma	All women over 40, African-Americans, or those with a family history of glaucoma

most studies indicate a benefit to combined hormone replacement therapy.

It is not clear how long a woman should take hormone replacement therapy or how long there is a benefit. Estrogen may be unsafe for women with a previous cancer of the breast or lining of the uterus, liver disease, or a history of blood clots in the lung related to hormone treatment (such as birth control pills) or pregnancy. For most women in their 50s or 60s, hormone replacement therapy offers benefits that they should seriously consider, but later in life the benefits may be outweighed by potential risks.

Sexuality

Women over the age of 70 years can and often do remain sexually active. The major cause of lack of sexual activity in older women is the lack of a male partner. Older women are able to experience sexual feelings and orgasm. Sexual responsiveness and desire may be affected in both sexes by depression, medical illness, or medications.

After menopause there is less lubrication in the vagina and the walls of the vagina become thinner and dryer. This can cause pain during intercourse. Estrogen can be effective in alleviating this problem whether it is taken by mouth in pill form or placed in the vagina as a cream or suppository.

Older couples should feel free to express their sexuality in ways that bring them pleasure. This may involve trying new positions that are less physically demanding or forms of sexual expression other than intercourse.

Substance Use

Tobacco and alcohol pose a risk to everyone. It is never too late to benefit from ending smoking or excess alcohol intake.

Among persons age 65–74, about 18 percent of women smoke. While this figure seems relatively low, it should be interpreted with caution. Because smoking increases the rate of death from coronary heart disease, stroke, and cancer, many people who smoke do not live long. Smoking is also a major contributor to lung disorders, such as emphysema and pneumonia, which can have devastating effects on the elderly.

Alcoholism is underrecognized late in life. The problem can arise after someone has suffered a loss or may have become established over years. The aged brain is more sensitive to alcohol, which in excess can cause confusion, falls, and injury. As it interacts with other drugs, alcohol can either interfere with their action or increase its own or the drugs' effects. This can pose a particular problem in the elderly because their rate of metabolism is slowed, making it more difficult to process the drugs in their systems.

Medications

Elderly people not only take more medications than any other age group, but also experience more adverse side effects. This is related to several factors, including exposure to a larger number of medications, drug interactions, errors in taking medication, delayed elimination of medications from the body, and a higher sensitivity to the medications themselves.

Because of changes that take place with age, ordinary doses of drugs remain within the body for longer periods than expected and can build up to high levels over time. In all age groups, the organs most responsible for removing drugs from the system are the kidney and liver.

Kidney function declines on the average with advancing age. When drugs are given that depend on the kidneys for processing, repeated use of the drug causes it to build up and become toxic. Commonly prescribed drugs in this category include digoxin, a heart medication; certain antibiotics; cimetidine (Tagamet), a drug given for peptic ulcer; and lithium, a drug given for certain psychiatric illnesses. Whenever these and other drugs are given to the elderly the doses must be carefully adjusted and monitored.

With advancing age the liver may be less able to process certain drugs. Examples of drugs processed by the liver include diazepam (Valium); flurazepam (Dalmane), a sleeping pill; and theophylline, an anti-asthma medication.

In addition to a lowered ability to remove drugs from their bodies, elderly people may be more sensitive to normal doses because the drug itself behaves differently. This effect is related to changes in various organs that occur with advancing age or with actual disease, which is more common in late life. Because disease often is not obvious in the elderly, the patient may have no symptoms until the stress of a medication is introduced.

The effects of a drug may be exaggerated in the elderly. For example, a normal dose of a sedative, intended to reduce anxiety or to have a calming effect, may produce sluggishness or confusion. Confusion is a side effect that can be produced in older people by a large number of drugs, probably because of the high prevalence of Alzheimer's and other forms of brain disease. In addition to sedatives, other medications that may produce confusion in elderly patients include sleeping pills, corticosteroids, arthritis medications, certain antidepressants, and some drugs given to lower blood pressure.

Although it is not always possible to predict the body's ability to process medication, cautious prescribing can help avoid overdose. Tests can be done to measure the amount of drug in the blood. These tests are available for many medications and are generally reliable. It is helpful to keep a list of *all* medications taken and their dosages, especially if they have been prescribed by more than one doctor, so the list can be reviewed by a doctor if there are problems.

HEALTH CONCERNS OF AGING

Early recognition and treatment of diseases that often occur in the elderly can help manage these disorders and keep them from progressing in some cases. The leading causes of death in women 65 years of age and older are cardiovascular disease, stroke, cancer, and pneumonia. Major causes of illness and disability include osteoporosis and arthritis, heart disease, falls, and hearing and vision impairment.

Cardiovascular System

The number one cause of death in both women and men is cardiovascular disease. This includes coronary heart disease, which causes the deaths of 236,000 women annually, as well as stroke and congestive heart failure—all of which increase dramatically with age. Coronary heart disease is the leading cause of death in women and outnumbers deaths in women caused by all cancers combined.

Coronary heart disease occurs in women about 10 years later than it does in men. Some believe this delay is due to the protection that estrogen provides against heart disease. Once a woman passes menopause, her risk begins to approach that of a man.

Coronary heart disease often is unrecognized in women. Women are diagnosed at later stages of disease than men are and are less often referred for diagnostic procedures. Women also tend to have surgical treatment, such as coronary artery bypass surgery, later in the course of the disease, which results in a higher rate of complications and death from the procedure. Women also have a greater degree of disability after heart attacks compared with men and are less likely to be referred for exercise and rehabilitation. The reasons for these differences are unclear.

The risk factors for coronary heart disease include diabetes, hypertension, cigarette smoking, abnormal cholesterol (see below), and family history. With the exception of family history, all of these factors can be controlled to lower the risk. Women with diabetes have a three-fold increased risk of heart attack, and it is a stronger factor for women than men. Diabetes can be controlled through a combination of diet, exercise, and medication to normalize blood sugar (glucose) level.

Hypertension, or high blood pressure greater than about 160 (millimeters of mercury) systolic pressure and 90 (millimeters of mercury) diastolic pressure, increases the risk of heart attack and stroke. The main form of hypertension affecting the elderly involves elevated systolic pressure with normal diastolic pressure. Although hypertension can have side effects and must be carefully monitored in the elderly, newer medications are very well tolerated.

There is no safe level of cigarette smoking. As few as one to four cigarettes per day increases the risk of heart attack. Smoking also affects other aspects of body function that increase the risk of stroke.

In women, high-density lipoprotein (HDL) cholesterol protects against heart attack, whereas low-density lipoprotein (LDL) cholesterol increases the risk. Estrogen increases HDL and decreases LDL. After menopause the ratio of LDL to HDL (or the ratio of total to HDL) cholesterol increases. Hormone replacement therapy appears to have a beneficial effect on cholesterol ratios and thus on the risk of heart disease. Women also can

PREVENTING CARDIOVASCULAR DISEASE

The following guidelines can help protect you against cardiovascular disease:

- Quit smoking.
- Have your blood pressure checked even if you feel well, and take medication if it is too high. Weight loss and reduction of salt intake are sometimes helpful.
- Be tested for diabetes if you have risk factors or symptoms and follow your doctor's recommendations regarding diet, exercise, and medication.
- Eat a low-fat, low-cholesterol diet and have your cholesterol levels checked.
- Exercise to increase cardiovascular fitness and help control hypertension and diabetes.
- Consider hormone replacement therapy.

often control cholesterol levels through diet.

A woman with a family member who had a heart attack before age 60 has a high risk of coronary heart disease. That relative could be a mother, father, or other first-degree relative. Women with this history should receive special attention in screening for coronary heart disease.

Heart attacks in women are often fatal. Prevention, early recognition, and treatment of coronary heart disease can prevent debility and premature death and are important aspects of a woman's general health care.

Musculoskeletal System

Approximately 50 percent of people age 65 or older have arthritis or rheumatism (pain and stiffness in some portion of the musculoskeletal system). They can be a source of discomfort and disability, representing common daily problems for many elderly (see Part III).

Arthritis

Arthritis is the most common inflammatory disease of joints, and 70 percent of those who have arthritis are women.

The most common cause of arthritis among the elderly is osteoarthritis, also known as degenerative joint disease. At least 40 million people in the United States have some evidence of the disease. Whereas osteoarthritis affects the knees or hands of older women, it more often affects the hips in older men. Both sexes may have pain in the spine. Osteoarthritis can be relieved with rest, muscle-strengthening exercise, medication, and use of an assistive device, such as a cane. In severe cases, surgery is an option. Hip and knee replacement surgery may be highly effective late in life. Advanced age alone is not a reason to avoid such surgery, and many very elderly people have benefited from surgery.

Two other forms of arthritis, gout and pseudogout, are more common with advancing age. Gout is caused by a buildup of uric acid crystals in the joints, most commonly the big toe or the knees. It causes redness, swelling, and pain in the affected joint. In postmenopausal women, gout is usually related to the use of diuretic medications that increase the level of uric acid in the blood. Stopping the diuretics or switching to different medication can reduce or stop the attacks. Pseudogout is not caused by uric acid crystals and is unrelated to diuretic use. It has symptoms similar to gout and is treated with medications used for arthritis.

Polymyalgia rheumatica (PMR) is a syndrome that includes achiness and severe stiffness that are worse in the morning. It affects people over age 50, two-thirds of whom are women. The disorder is diagnosed by a blood test and treated with corticosteroids, usually for about a year.

Temporal arthritis may accompany PMR but is a more serious form of the disease. It is an inflammation of the arteries that lie on the forehead, and the symptoms are headaches, dizziness, and blurred or suddenly lost vision. If treatment with corticosteroids is not begun right away, permanent loss of vision may occur.

Osteoporosis

Bone loss, which can result in osteoporosis, occurs as a normal part of aging. Rate of bone loss accelerates in women for a few years after menopause, when fractures linked to bone loss begin to increase dramatically. Among people over age 65, eight times as many women as men have spinal fractures due to bone loss. By age 90, at least 30 percent of women have had fractured hips, the most severe form of osteoporotic fracture, which often results in disability and serious health problems. Osteoporosis also leads to weakening and collapse of the spinal bones, resulting in forward curving of the spine (see Figure 1.1). The best treatment of osteoporosis is early prevention through diet, exercise, and hormone replacement therapy.

Osteomalacia

A condition that also causes bone fragility in the elderly, osteomalacia often coexists with osteoporosis and has similar symptoms. Osteomalacia is reversible, how-

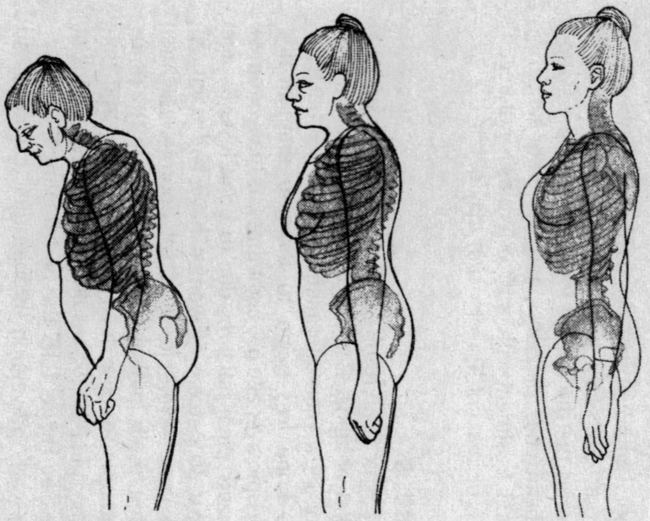

Figure 1.1 Spinal Curvature
Progressive forward curvature ("kyphosis") occurs in women at high risk of developing spinal osteoporosis.

ever, and osteoporosis is not. Osteomalacia is usually caused by vitamin D deficiency. Vitamin D controls the body's use of calcium and is found in certain foods, such as deep sea fish and fortified milk products. Elderly men and women who lack exposure to sunlight are at risk of vitamin D deficiency. This problem can occur in cold climates or when people are housebound or reside in nursing homes. Even though the condition is treated with vitamin D, excessive doses may cause illness and should be avoided.

Accidents

Although spinal fractures can occur without trauma, most fractures in the elderly occur as the result of a fall. As many as one-third of older adults fall at least once a year, and these falls often result in fractures. Falls can be caused by a number of preventable problems, such as being distracted, slipping, or stumbling. Among the elderly, most falls occur indoors. Falls also occur due to medical problems, such as overmedication, strokes, TIAs (a type of stroke), heart rhythm disturbances, or general weakness or illness. An elderly person should be carefully evaluated after a fall to detect any problems. People with physical disabilities should receive physical therapy and training in the use of devices such as canes, walkers, or leg braces. The home should be evaluated for potential hazards, such as slippery rugs or shaky handrails, and made as safe as possible.

Memory Loss

With increasing age, there is increasing risk of developing problems with memory. When memory loss is severe enough to interfere with work or social functioning, and when there is an accompanying impairment in intellectual function, the condition is known as dementia. The most common form of dementia is Alzheimer's disease, a condition that is more common in women than in men. The higher prevalence in women may be due to the fact that the disease usually appears late in life, when there are more women than men.

Alzheimer's disease is not an epidemic. Recent publicity reflects scientific scrutiny of a condition that once was once called "senility" and was thought to be due to "hardening of the arteries." With increasing awareness of the true causes of "senility," more cases of Alzheimer's disease have been correctly diagnosed. In addition, as more and more people survive into old age, more cases of Alzheimer's disease, as well as other forms of dementia, will be identified.

Older men and women without signs of dementia commonly complain of memory loss. For example, people often complain of walking into a room but forgetting the reason they are there. This problem occurs at all ages, however, and can be due to trivial factors like distraction. This sort of memory lapse is less likely to create anxiety in a younger individual than it is in an elderly one, who might be concerned that it is a sign of Alzheimer's disease. Certain changes are common with age that may be quite normal including slower speed in processing visual, auditory, and sensory information and difficulty finding words, especially proper nouns. True dementia, however, is common only among people who survive into their eighties and beyond.

Most people who seek medical attention on their own because of memory loss are functioning normally and may not be at high risk of developing Alzheimer's disease. People brought to the attention of physicians by concerned family or friends, however, often have already developed a significant problem.

Memory loss always should be evaluated because it can be linked with a number of disorders. If a significant change in a person's memory and mental abilities has taken place within hours, days, or weeks, medical attention is required right away. Rapid changes in memory are usually due to overmedication or serious medical illness.

When memory loss slowly progresses over a year or more, a reversible cause rarely exists. In all cases, a careful medical evaluation and regular follow-up are required.

People with dementia have a higher risk of being injured. They also may have other medical problems, such as an infection, that makes the condition worse. A wide variety of medical illnesses may have the symptoms of sudden worsening of dementia, lethargy, incontinence, and lowered intake of food and fluid. Such situations require immediate medical attention.

The Immune System

People in later life are more prone to certain infections. This may be partly related to changes in the immune system that protects the body from disease. The function of these cells combating disease declines with age. Some elderly may be less able to produce antibodies in response to vaccines for pneumonia or influenza, which protect them from these diseases. Despite this, vaccinations are very effective in most elderly people and we strongly urge receiving them as recommended (see "Routine Care for Women 65 Years and Older"). Two important infections that occur among the elderly are pneumonia and urinary tract infections.

Pneumonia

Pneumonia that is not acquired in an institution is most often due to the bacterium pneumococcus, which can be prevented with a vaccine. Chronically ill or disabled elderly, especially those in institutions or who have just undergone surgery, are also at increased risk for pneumonia caused by other bacteria. Although the vaccine does not protect them, the infection can be treated with antibiotics. If treatment is given, usually the patient's underlying health rather than a specific type of bacterium determines whether she will recover.

Immunizations

Vaccines make people immune to a disease. Immunization with pneumococcal vaccine is recommended for all people age 65 and older. Since a variety of bacterial pneumonias can occur as a complication of influenza, and since death due to pneumonia increases with age, all persons over the age of 65 should receive an annual influenza vaccine shot. It must be given every year because the virus that causes influenza is constantly changing. This vaccine prevents infection caused only by influenza virus, which is why immunized people can still get flulike illnesses not due to the virus.

Diphtheria and tetanus are potentially serious illnesses that can be prevented by immunization. Although these diseases do not occur frequently today, most deaths caused by them occur among the elderly, who are the least protected for several reasons. Most of today's elderly did not receive standard immunizations because such programs did not exist during their school years. Women are the group at highest risk because most women did not receive immunizations given through the military. Even if a person did receive the vaccine, its effectiveness is reduced over time. Elderly people uncertain of their immunization histories should have a series of three shots in six months.

Blood

Iron deficiency can be a cause of anemia in older adults of both sexes. In the United States, many foods are fortified with iron, so iron deficiency usually does not result from lack of iron in the diet. Instead, iron deficiency in the United States is almost always due to blood loss. Among the elderly, blood loss can be silent and may result from either a peptic ulcer (an ulcer of the stomach or upper intestine) or colon cancer.

Because there may be no signs or symptoms of blood loss, and only small amounts can be lost over time, iron deficiency may be the first sign of a serious disease. Iron deficiency usually can be detected by a blood test; and other tests may confirm the results. Older people who are taking vitamin supplements should select products that do not contain iron because supplemental iron might mask an iron deficiency due to silent blood loss.

A stomach condition called atrophic gastritis that occurs with aging can interfere with the body's ability to absorb B-12. Vitamin B-12 deficiency can produce anemia and neurologic problems, but it is uncertain how often this occurs in the elderly today. There are some simple and very sensitive tests to measure vitamin B-12 in the blood. Use of these tests has led to the detection of low levels in many elderly, but the link with disease is not clear. In theory, vitamin B-12 deficiency can produce disease of the nervous system, including psychiatric syndromes, memory loss, and spinal degeneration, even before anemia occurs. A number of healthy older people have low vitamin B-12 levels, and low levels do occur more commonly in patients with dementia, but B-12 supplementation rarely restores memory. Low B-12 levels should be treated with B-12 injections, or in some cases pills, as determined by a physician.

Atrophic gastritis is a condition that is often treated with B-12 injections, but consult your physician.

People with chronic illness often have what is called anemia of chronic disease. This form of relatively mild anemia usually requires no specific treatment.

The Urinary System

Urinary tract disorders often occur in older women and can be related to a problem in the system or in an underlying disorder. Symptoms can be caused by urinary incontinence, infection of urine, or structural problems. Urinary incontinence can have a major impact on women and their families and be a source of embarrassment, loss of mobility, and low self-esteem. Available treatments can be very effective even in women in very late life.

Urinary Tract Infections

Although these infections are very common in women of all ages, a large number of elderly women have recurrent bladder infections. This may have to do with changes in the bladder and surrounding tissues that are exposed to bacteria. While as many as one-half of older woman have signs of bacteria in their urine, the condition should not be treated unless symptoms are present because overtreatment with antibiotics can lead to the development of antibiotic-resistant strains of bacteria. Vaginal estrogen cream can help prevent urinary tract infection in postmenopausal women.

Urinary Incontinence

Urinary incontinence is the involuntary loss of urine. The most common causes are "unstable bladder" and "stress incontinence," which often coexist. In unstable bladder, symptoms may include urgency, which is the strong desire to void (or urinate), accompanied by the fear of leakage, and frequency, which is defined as voiding more than seven times in 24 hours or every two hours. Another symptom is nocturia, which is being awakened from sleep by the urge to void two or more times per night. Symptoms can be related to another medical problem or to the use of medications.

Stress incontinence consists of leakage of small amounts of urine after a cough, sneeze, or any maneuver that increases the abdominal pressure exerted on the bladder. Most often stress incontinence results from the relaxation of the supporting tissues of the urethra, bladder, and other pelvic organs. These changes are thought to be related to childbirth, but many older women who never have given birth are affected probably because of age-related changes in supporting tissues. After menopause, these tissues become stretched and weakened because of a lack of estrogen. (See Figure 1.2).

KEGEL EXERCISES

These exercises can strengthen the muscles of the pelvic floor surrounding the urethra, vagina, and anus. A doctor or nurse should show you how to do them. The muscles should be contracted and held for about 3 seconds, then released for 3 seconds, 12–15 times in a row, five or six times a day. As an alternate method, you can perform 10–12 contractions each for 10 seconds three times a day. The exercises should not be done while voiding. At least 40 exercises per day must be done to benefit from the program.

Other Causes of Incontinence

Hospitalized women may experience temporary urinary incontinence after surgery or if they are chronically bedridden. Mild incontinence may be brought on or preexisting incontinence may temporarily worsen as a result of an acute bladder infection, which causes irritation to the bladder or urethra; however, older women often have bladder infections when symptoms are not present. The sudden onset of urinary incontinence may result from a state of confusion, which should receive immediate medical attention because it could be a sign of serious illness.

Patients with dementia often have urinary incontinence. It is uncertain if the incontinence is directly related to a specific problem in the brain or due to confusion about the location or method of toileting, or both. Standard incontinence therapy does not work in these patients. Toileting on schedule—for example, every 2–4 hours, depending on the woman's needs—may help keep her dry. Incontinence garments, or diapers, can be used, although they are not acceptable to some women. Adult diapers must be changed frequently and special attention should be given to hygiene. A catheter, a tube placed and left in the bladder to drain the urine into a bag, should be avoided because it may lead to bladder infection.

Incontinence can be caused by medicine, especially in older women who may already have abnormal function of the bladder or urethra. The most common offenders are diuretics, especially potent ones such as furosemide. If this drug must be taken, it is often helpful to take it during the time of the day that best suits the woman; for instance, she could take it when she is at home and has easy access to a bathroom. Other medications that can produce incontinence include prazosin (Minipress) or terazosin (Hytrin), which are used to control blood pressure but which weaken the urethra and allow urine to leak.

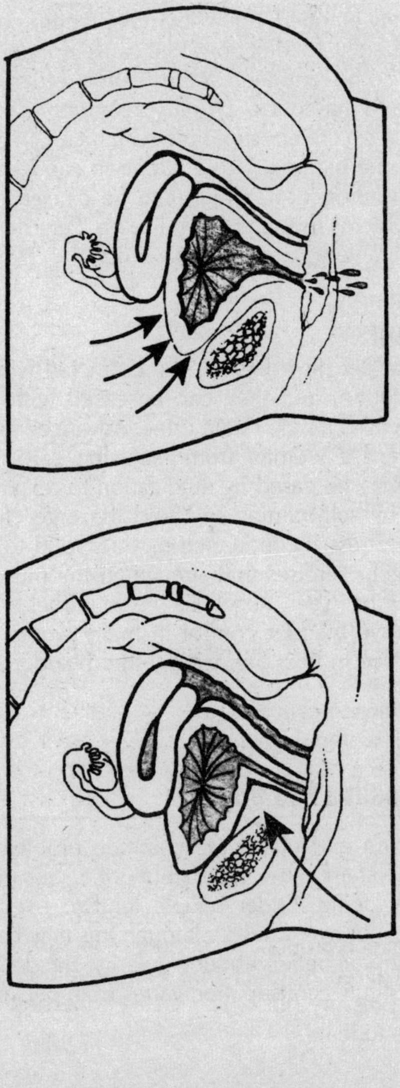

Figure 1.2 Stress Urinary Incontinence

Normal anatomy—no urine leakage under pressure.

Abnormal anatomy—patulous urethra and loss of sharp bladder angle lead to urine leakage under pressure.

Medications can also cause retention of urine and "overflow incontinence." Because the bladder is not completely emptied, the woman has feelings of urgency and frequency. Medications that cause urinary retention include some antidepressants, some older antihistamines, and narcotics. Urinary retention can also be caused by severe constipation, which can compress the outlet of the bladder. Urine retention can be related to bladder malfunction, which can be caused by neurologic problems or underlying disease. Persistent urinary retention is very rare in older women.

Treatment

Some bladder disorders can be corrected with surgery or medication, and they can be eased with exercises and devices that help retain urine. Advanced age should not prevent a woman from receiving care. Unstable bladder may be eased by medication to relax the bladder and by self-training to "hold the urge" for longer intervals. Stress incontinence may respond to estrogen or to Kegel exercises that strengthen the muscles controlling urine (see "Kegel Exercises"). These exercises can improve bladder control in many women but are less effective in later life, when other bladder problems coexist.

The Digestive System

Constipation and ulcers are common problems of the digestive system in the elderly but not necessarily a part of normal aging. Older people tend to use laxatives more than younger adults, although this may have to do with traditional beliefs about regularity. The definition of what constitutes constipation varies from person to person. As with any age group, a change in bowel habits should be evaluated by a doctor.

Constipation

Constipation often occurs in elderly people who are immobilized, such as those who are homebound or live in nursing homes. These people tend to get constipated because of lack of exercise, decreased intake of fiber and fluids, medical problems that can interfere with bowel function, and certain medications. Medications that cause constipation include calcium channel blocking agents, calcium supplements, aluminum-containing antacids, narcotics, and certain antidepressants or related compounds.

Treatment of constipation consists of physical exercise, increasing the intake of fluid, changing medications if possible, and eating food high in fiber. Excess fiber intake (as found in fiber-containing cookies) should be avoided, however, especially in bedbound patients, because it may worsen the problem. Laxative abuse, longstanding daily use of laxatives, may damage the nerve supply in the bowel and make constipation worse. Laxatives should be used, however, in patients with physical limitations who are prone to fecal impaction. In this extreme form of constipation there may be little or no bowel movement.

Ulcers

Ulcers can occur in the duodenum (upper small intestine) or the stomach (gastric ulcers). Ulcers in the duodenum are more common, but the risk of gastric ulcers increases with age. Older people are at a higher risk of gastric ulcer because of thinning of the lining of the stomach. They also use aspirinlike medications more frequently, particularly nonsteroidal anti-inflammatory agents (NSAIDs), such as ibuprofen. Although these medications relieve arthritis and other painful conditions, they may disrupt the stomach lining and produce an array of ulcer and ulcerlike conditions.

Occasional use of NSAIDs is usually not a problem, and some products are available without a prescription. Repeated use of even moderate doses can pose a major risk among the elderly, however. It is best to treat painful conditions with other medications, such as acetaminophen (Tylenol and other brands) or, if pain is severe, narcotic-containing preparations. When prolonged use of NSAIDs is required, the woman should be monitored closely by a physician with periodic checks of stool and blood samples, including iron levels. Ulcer disease is more likely to be silent in the elderly and may produce painless bleeding. Blood loss can be slow and steady, which can be detected on a routine stool exam or blood test, or it can be massive. Certain patients may benefit from antiulcer medications. It is now known that bacteria play a role in ulcer disease, but they appear to play little or no role in NSAID-induced stomach ulcers.

Duodenal ulcers are almost always benign and heal readily with proper treatment. Approximately 5 percent of gastric ulcers are cancers, and this rate is somewhat higher among older people. It is essential, therefore, that gastric ulcers be biopsied initially and then reevaluated after a course of treatment to be sure they have healed.

Skin

Some changes in skin occur with aging, while others are due to damage from the sun and other environmental factors. With normal aging, changes occur in collagen, an important protein in the skin. Sun damage is usually confined to exposed areas and can be shown by comparing these areas (forehead, neck, hands, and forearms) with skin protected from the sun (lower back, abdomen, and buttocks.) These differences are most pronounced in light-skinned individuals, especially those who have had a great deal of exposure to the sun throughout their lives. The differences are least obvious in people with deeply pigmented skin. Solar damage causes wrinkles, freckles, precancerous lesions called actinic keratoses, and skin cancer.

Normal aging results in skin sagging but not wrinkling or developing other problems caused by environmental skin damage. Normal aging causes a loss of elastic tissue, changes in collagen, and thinning of the upper layers of the skin. Body fat is redistributed from the layer immediately beneath the skin to the deeper layers, and from the extremities, face, and neck to the trunk. This redistribution gives the appearance of skin sagging and wrinkling.

Tretinoin (Retin-A) is a medication used for acne that is available as a cream and appears to reverse some of the effects of environmental skin damage. There is no evidence, however, that it reverses age-related skin changes.

Use of sun blocks and reducing sunlight exposure can prevent premature aging of the skin and can reduce the risk of skin cancer. Sunlight is important to the production of vitamin D, however, so exposure should not be avoided entirely. Sunlight also may have an effect on mood, and its role in alleviating seasonal affective disorder, a condition in which depression is linked to lack of exposure to daylight, is being explored.

Skin cancer occurs more often with increasing age. The most common form in late life is basal cell carcinoma. Unlike other forms of skin cancer, basal cell carcinoma rarely spreads to distant sites. It grows very slowly and is almost always curable. The tumor can affect adjoining areas, however, and should be removed without delay.

EXERCISE AND AGING

Exercise continues to be important in later life. It improves cardiovascular fitness, may help slow the bone loss that occurs with osteoporosis, helps lower blood sugar in people with diabetes, and helps control cholesterol. In addition, exercise promotes weight loss, muscle strength, and a general feeling of well-being. Studies suggest that lack of exercise contributes to frailness and weakness in elderly people.

Exercise can promote cardiovascular fitness by increasing the efficiency of the heart's function. As the body works, it requires more oxygen and the heart beats faster. Exercise increases the body's ability to use oxygen, which enables a person to exercise more without feeling tired. Exercise must reach a certain level to provide this benefit. The target heart rate can be a guide to reaching a level of exercise that provides cardiovascular fitness. However, this guide should be used cautiously late in life, when silent heart disease may exist.

Some forms of exercise strengthen the back muscles making them less prone to injury and strain. Other types of exercise help prevent bone loss by strengthening the bones and keeping them from becoming brittle. To provide bone strength, weight-bearing exercises are best. For instance, walking and lifting weights are forms of exercise that are weight bearing, whereas swimming and cycling, although they are good forms of cardiovascular conditioning, are much less likely to prevent bone loss.

An older woman who has not been exercising should consult her physician before beginning an exercise program. She must begin a new exercise program slowly and carefully. Physical changes may increase the risk of injury, and heart disease may be present but not apparent.

Older women should choose a form of exercise that is safe and comfortably within their physical capabilities. Jogging and high-impact aerobics can cause injury at any age but such exercises pose additional risk of injury to older people. Better options for cardiovascular fitness include walking, low-impact aerobics, and swimming.

People with severe physical impairments may still improve their level of fitness by doing limited exercise in the sitting position. Elderly patients who become ill and need to be hospitalized or confined to bed for even a few days suffer rapid deterioration of their physical condition because they cannot move around. This can be avoided by maintaining some level of physical activity during and after illness, which also lowers the risk of bed sores (pressure ulcers), pneumonia, and blood clots.

For a woman entering or past the age of menopause, exercising may be the single best thing she can do for her emotional and physical health. Whether or not she takes estrogen replacement, the active postmenopausal woman has a much better chance of keeping her heart healthy, her bones strong, and her body fit than her more sedentary sisters (Figure 1.3). The woman over 60 who exercises at least 30 minutes three times per week has the heart, lungs, and muscles of a woman ten years younger.

It can actually be dangerous to your health *not* to exercise. A serious concern for the older woman is the threat of osteoporosis, a degenerative bone disorder. Women reach a peak bone mass at around age 30, after

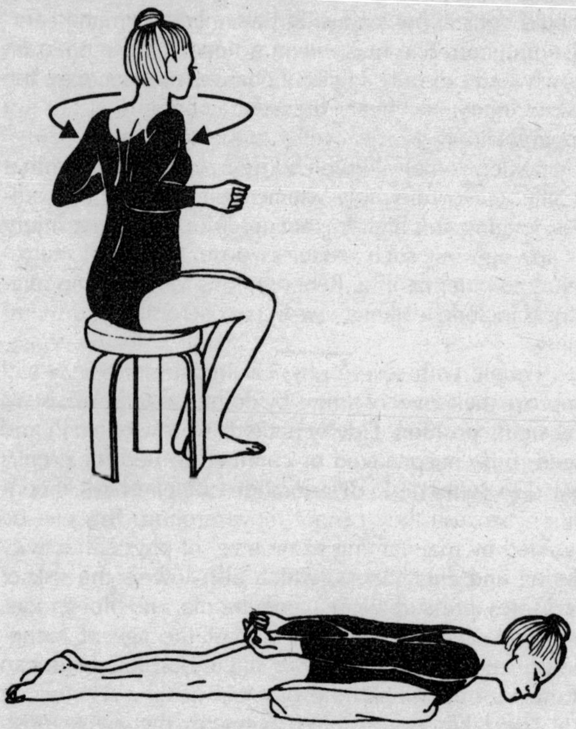

Figure 1.3 Back-Strengthening Exercises.
Strengthening your back muscles can help avoid the back pain that often accompanies aging.
Top: To strengthen the trapezius muscles in the upper back and shoulders, sit with your back straight and your feet on the floor. With your arms relaxed and bent, pull back your shoulders as far as they will go.
Bottom: Lie facedown with a cushion under your hips and torso, your arms at your sides, and your legs straight. Lift your head and feet off the floor at the same time and hold, then relax and repeat.

which bone gradually decreases until menopause, when a rapid decrease occurs if replacement hormones are not administered. Along with nutritional factors (not eating adequate dietary calcium), lack of exercise may be an important promoter of accelerated bone loss.

In addition, women well past the age of menopause may be able to slow the rate of bone loss by performing weight-bearing exercises. Remember, even if you are returning to exercise after a period of inactivity, you are not starting from zero. Muscles may in fact have "memory." Being active in any way will do a lot to improve overall health in the later years.

Since older joints become stiff and inflexible there may be a need to do a longer warm-up and modify your exercise—perhaps by doing fewer repetitions. Work at your own decreased target heart rate. And always be alert to any danger signs: lightheadedness, chest pain, or shortness of breath. In terms of specific exercises, calisthenics promote flexibility, weightlifting promotes muscle strength, brisk walking is beneficial and convenient; and stationary bicycling and swimming strengthen the heart muscles. Jogging may not be a good choice: the jogger's foot lands with a force equal to several times body weight, which can injure older bones, tendons, ligaments, and joints.

Again, it's never too late to start exercising. A 1987 survey on exercise, diet, and bone loss in the *Journal of the American Geriatrics Society* found that sedentary nursing home residents in their eighties experienced more than a 4 percent increase in density of the forearm bone when they performed mild exercises three times a week for three years. A group of nonexercisers underwent a 2.5 percent decline in bone density over the same time period.

Exercise will also help you maintain your weight or lose weight, even as your metabolism slows as you age. Not only will staying fit directly help you avoid developing serious diseases, such as diabetes and heart disease, but by exercising you will look and feel younger and more energetic. You may find that exercising alleviates some menopausal symptoms such as annoying hot flashes, and that your complexion looks and feels younger as more blood is pumped into the tiny capillaries that feed the skin. Improved circulation will also help your digestive system stay healthy and keep your immune system strong.

It's no wonder that the National Institutes of Health refer to exercise as "the most effective anti-aging pill ever discovered."

No one has found the fountain of youth—but you can certainly increase your odds and live longer and better by exercising. Staying physically fit should be a lifetime commitment.

MENOPAUSE

At menopause, a woman stops menstruating and her ovaries no longer produce estrogen. The average age at the last menstrual period is 51 or 52. This natural process begins several years before, as a woman's ovaries produce less and less estrogen. The lack of estrogen can produce a number of effects:

- Hot flashes or flushes can occur. These are sudden feelings of heat that spread over the body, often accompanied by a flushed face and sweating. They appear at any time without warning and are most troublesome at night when they can interfere with sleep.
- Vaginal tissue may become dryer, thinner, and less flexible. This can result in painful intercourse, urinary tract problems, or sagging of pelvic organs

because the tissues that support them lose their elasticity.

- Osteoporosis, or bone loss, can cause bones to become thin and brittle. Supplemental estrogen can help guard against it, as can a diet high in calcium, regular exercise, and stopping smoking.
- Cardiovascular disease becomes more of a risk for women after menopause because estrogen no longer gives them natural protection from heart attack and stroke.
- Emotional changes, such as mood swings, irritability, and depression, can accompany menopause, but these symptoms are more likely related to insomnia caused by hot flashes at night than to the lack of estrogen.

Not all women have all of these symptoms and they are not always long lasting. You can continue to have a full and healthy life for many years beyond menopause. Some of the symptoms of menopause can be eased through diet and exercise. Others can be relieved by replacing the estrogen no longer produced by the ovaries. Hormone replacement therapy can relieve the symptoms of menopause, in addition to lowering the risk of heart disease and osteoporosis.

Estrogen is given along with the hormone progestin (a synthetic version of the natural hormone progesterone) to protect against endometrial cancer, a risk when estrogen is taken alone. Estrogen by itself causes the lining of the uterus to overgrow and increases the risk of cancer of the endometrium. Progestin is taken with estrogen to oppose it and keep the lining of the endometrium in check. In fact, taking progestin with estrogen actually lowers the risk of cancer to less than that of a woman not taking hormone therapy.

Estrogen is processed through the liver and affects

the levels of cholesterol. Estrogen increases high-density cholesterol (the good cholesterol) and lowers low-density cholesterol (the bad cholesterol), thus reducing the risk of heart disease. Without estrogen, a woman's risk of heart disease approaches that of a man by age 65.

Women are at higher risk of osteoporosis because they have less bone mass than men to begin with and because they tend to have less calcium stored in their bones. Thus, when they lose the protective effect of estrogen, the natural process of bone loss speeds up so they are losing bone faster than it is being replaced.

Osteoporosis and cardiovascular disease do not have symptoms in their early stages as they are conditions that develop over time. Hormone replacement therapy to prevent symptoms of menopause also helps prevent these conditions. To provide long-term protection, the therapy must be taken long term.

Hormone replacement therapy is not for everyone. It is not recommended for women who have had breast cancer, endometrial cancer, or liver cancer. The link between breast cancer and hormone replacement therapy is still not clear. There may be a slight increase in a woman's chance of developing breast cancer if she has been taking hormones for more than 15 years.

Hormone replacement therapy can have other side effects. The progestin causes monthly bleeding or spotting, which can be bothersome. Other side effects include breast tenderness, fluid retention, swelling, mood changes, and pelvic cramping. Because of the side effects, some women choose to take estrogen alone. These women should be monitored carefully for abnormal bleeding. Their doctors may suggest that an endometrial biopsy be performed so a small amount of tissue can be examined.

Women who prefer not to take hormone replacement therapy can obtain relief of symptoms and help prevent bone loss and heart disease in other ways. To facilitate decisions about hormones, women should have a fasting cholesterol and a bone density test. Estrogen cream, used in the vagina, can treat vaginal dryness. A balanced diet rich in calcium and low in fat, regular exercise, and avoiding alcohol and tobacco can help reduce the rate of bone loss and protect against heart disease. Regardless of age or whether they are taking hormone replacement therapy, women should continue to have regular pelvic exams, mammograms, and Pap tests after they reach menopause.

Menopause and Sexuality

During menopause, a woman's ovaries stop producing the hormone estrogen. This can lead to changes that affect her sexual function. The main change is vaginal dryness. Lack of vaginal lubrication can make sex painful. Low levels of estrogen may also cause the walls of the vagina to thin and be more prone to sexual discomfort and injury. This can be corrected through estrogen replacement therapy. The hormone is taken as a pill or absorbed through a patch. Locally applied vaginal cream can also be used.

Women do not lose their sexual drive during or after menopause. Most women continue to enjoy a sexually fulfilling life throughout their later years. Factors that could interfere with this include health and relationship problems, availability of partners, and emotional concerns that may accompany menopause.

The nature of a woman's sexual activity may change as she ages. She may take longer to become aroused and may need more stimulation to have an orgasm. Some older women have fewer vaginal contractions during orgasm. Older men may have difficulty getting or keeping an erection. As their sexual needs change with age, couples may move their focus away from the traditional genital-focused approach to other forms of sexual pleasure. These may include manual stimulation, oral-genital stimulation, and rubbing the external genitals against each other. For many couples, although the physical form of their lovemaking may change, the intensity, satisfaction and frequency remain unchanged.

Older couples who are not comfortable with creating diverse experiences of sexual behavior may find their sexual activity limited. At some point, couples may be content to stop having sex. If both partners are comfortable with this situation, it does not have a negative effect on their relationship.

PART II

The Brain and Nervous System

Carolyn Barley Britton, M.D., M.S.

Among the most complex of the body mechanisms, the nervous system is responsible for thought, intellect, language, movement, sensation, and certain workings of other organ systems. Because the brain and nerves together act as a kind of control center for the body and its functions, any disorders of the systems may have far-reaching effects in different parts of the body.

Nervous system disorders can be *primary,* that is due to intrinsic dysfunction of the components of the nervous system. Or they can be *secondary,* that is, due to systemic illness, nutritional deficiency, exposure to toxic substances, or injury, among other causes. Neurological symptoms or disorders are present in 10 percent of outpatients, 12 percent of emergency room patients, and 15 percent of hospitalized patients.

STRUCTURE AND FUNCTION OF THE NERVOUS SYSTEM

The nervous system is comprised of several subsystems:

- The *central nervous system,* which consists of the brain and spinal cord (see Fig. 2.1).
- The *peripheral or neuromuscular system* comprising the cranial and peripheral nerves, emanating from the brain and spinal cord respectively; the neuromuscular junction (the synapse or connection of peripheral nerves to muscles); and muscle (see Fig. 2.2).
- The *autonomic nervous system,* which consists of sympathetic and parasympathetic fibers that arise from the spinal cord and terminate on internal organs such as the heart, gastrointestinal tract, bladder, and sex organs. This system affects heart

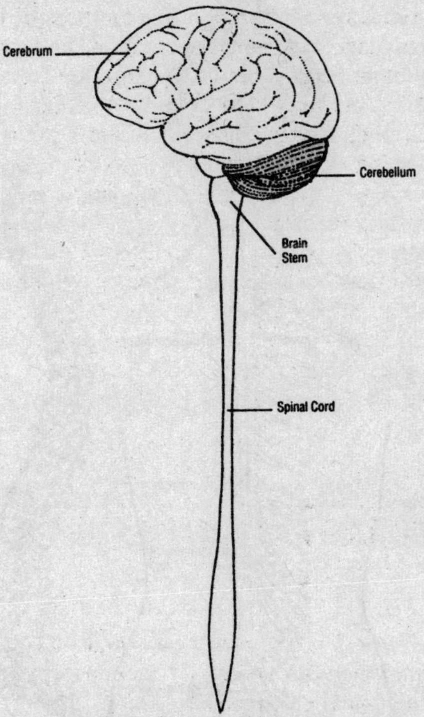

Figure 2.1 Functions of the Nervous System
The spinal cord conducts nerve signals between the body and the brain. The brain stem, at the juncture of the spinal cord and the brain, is responsible for breathing, heart function, and sleep cycles. Just above the brain stem, the cerebellum manages coordination, balance, and posture. Above the cerebellum is the limbic system, which controls primitive urges (such as self-preservation, emotions, moods, some senses, and certain bodily functions such as reproduction). The cerebrum is the largest and most highly developed part of the human brain. It allows impulses, thoughts, and ideas. The cerebrum is divided into two parts or lobes, each of which is responsible for different functions (see Fig. 2.3).

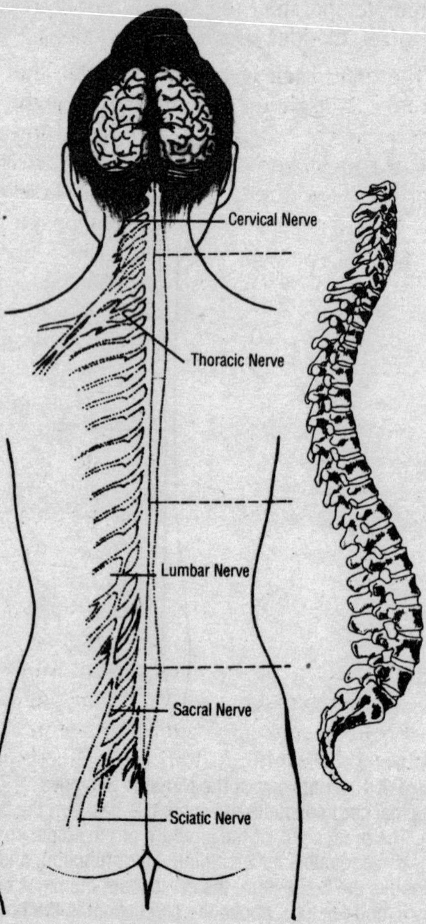

Figure 2.2 The Peripheral Nervous System
Nerves extend from the spinal cord between each vertebra in the spinal column and bring sensation to various parts of the body. The nerves are identified by the region of the spine from which they arise.

rate, temperature regulation, blood pressure, and bowel, bladder, and sexual functions.

The brain itself is a complex organ that consists of cerebral hemispheres controlling thought, language, memory, spatial orientation, sensation, and movement. Its basal ganglia and the cerebellum are responsible for motor tone, postural control, and coordination; the brain stem controls consciousness, respiration, heart rate, temperature regulation, and cranial nerve function (see Fig. 2.3). Motor and sensory fibers also pass through the brain stem, ascending from the spinal cord or descending from the cerebral hemispheres.

The brain and spinal cord are bathed in cerebrospinal fluid (CSF), which extracts nutrients such as glucose from the blood to supply the cells of the nervous system and removes cellular wastes. For protection, both are covered by three membranes and encased in bony structures, the skull and vertebral column, respectively. Nerves issuing from the brain stem supply the special sense organs (eyes, ears, nose), the facial muscles, and muscles of chewing, speech, and swallowing (cranial nerves). From the spinal cord, nerves emanate to supply muscles of the limbs and trunk (peripheral nerves) and internal organs (autonomic nerves). The vertebral column surrounding the spinal cord is a segmented structure resembling interlocking blocks separated by a gelatinous material, the intervertebral disc, which is held in place by strong, fibrous bands (see Fig. 2.4). Ligaments help to maintain the stability of the column and allow for movement.

The basic functional unit of the nervous system is the *neuron,* or nerve cell. Because neurons do not divide and have limited regenerative capacity, their loss may result in permanent neurological disability. Billions of neurons in the brain and spinal cord communicate with each other—by contacts or *synapses*—and with the

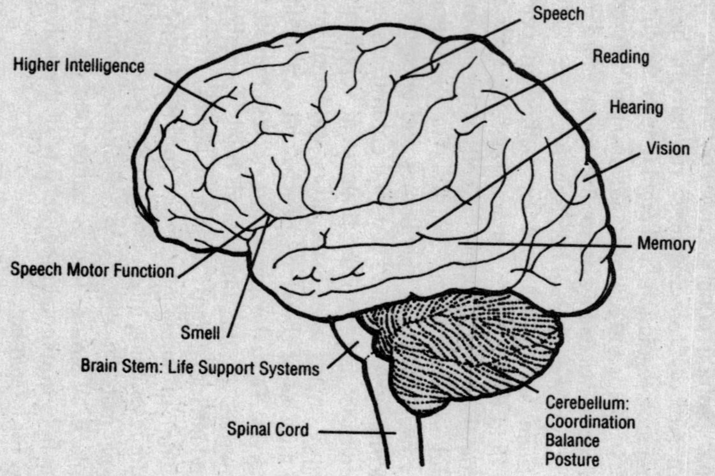

Figure 2.3 The Brain
Different parts of the brain control various functions in the body.

muscles and internal organs. The spinal cord and sense organs also send impulses to the brain, generating neural activity responsible for all aspects of human behavior. Impulses from neurons in the cerebral hemispheres of the brain are sent through branching nerve fibers called *axons* that terminate on other neurons in the basal ganglia, brain stem, or spinal cord. Messages are relayed via their axons to the cranial or spinal nerves (see Fig. 2.5). Some axons are several feet long, stretching from the brain to the lower spinal cord, and many are covered by a sheath called *myelin* that enhances the speed of conduction of nerve impulses. Other supporting cells in the nervous system, called *glia,* modulate neural activity and provide nutritional support. When a nerve impulse reaches the end of an axon, it causes the release of specific chemicals, the "messengers" of nerve activity.

The nervous system is dependent on a continuous supply of oxygen and glucose delivered by the blood. Because the brain has no capacity to store oxygen or glucose, interruption of blood flow for a few minutes may result in permanent neurological damage. The brain alone receives approximately 20 percent of the cardiac output of blood. The major blood vessels to the brain are the two internal carotid arteries and the two vertebral arteries. The carotid arteries supply the hemispheres of the brain, and the vertebral arteries supply the brain stem and cerebellum. The two circulations meet in a structure at the base of the brain called the *circle of Willis.*

Disorders of the brain and nervous system can cause various conditions.

1. Cell death or dysfunction (stroke, Alzheimer's disease, Parkinson's disease) due to loss of blood supply or oxygen, degenerative disease, trauma, infection, tumor, or toxins
2. Loss of critical support structures such as myelin,

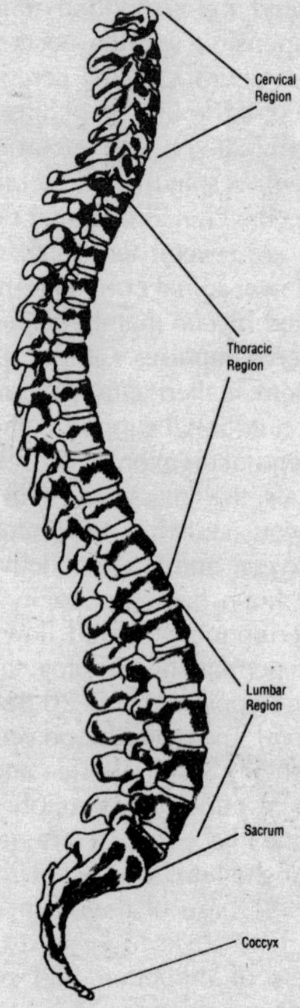

Figure 2.4 The Spinal Column
The spinal cord is enclosed with the 33 vertebrae, bones that make up the spinal column: seven cervical, twelve thoracic, five lumbar, five sacral, and four that form the coccyx at the base of the spine.

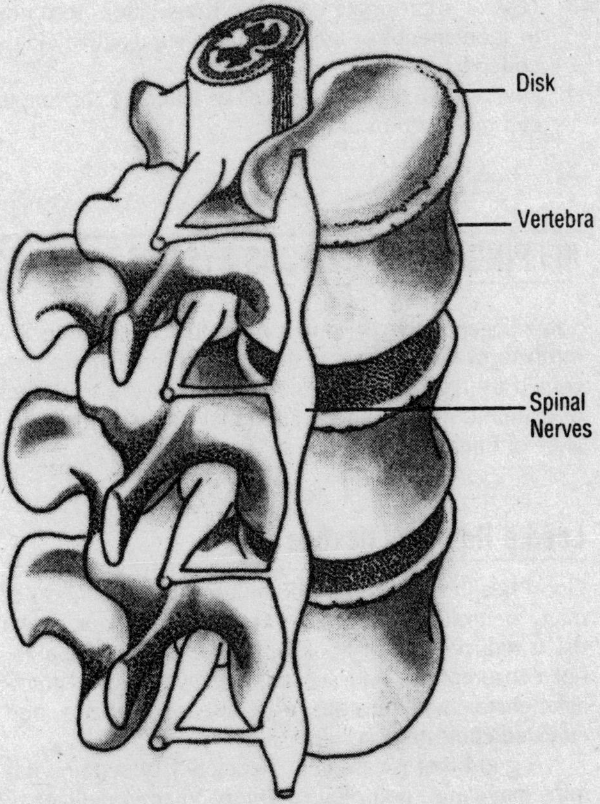

Figure 2.5 The Spinal Cord
The spinal cord is protected by the vertebral column, which is made up of interlocking bones called vertebrae. Intervertebral discs provide cushioning between the vertebrae, which are connected by ligaments that allow movement of the spinal column.

resulting in slowing of nerve impulse transmission (multiple sclerosis) and, if massive, cell death
3. Loss of appropriate cell-to-cell regulation, resulting in spontaneous or inappropriate neural activity (e.g., epileptic seizures)
4. Loss of critical nutrients such as vitamins, leading to cell malfunction or death.

KEEPING YOUR NERVOUS SYSTEM HEALTHY

Some degenerative or genetic neurological disorders are intrinsic to the nervous system, but others can be prevented by regular health maintenance, early treatment of systemic illness, good nutritional habits, and avoidance of injury.

Lead a Healthy Lifestyle

Good health habits are important for the prevention of many neurological diseases. For example, your stroke risk is reduced by not smoking, avoiding excessive alcohol consumption, and seeking effective medical management of hypertension, heart disease, diabetes, and elevated cholesterol.

A good diet is essential. Deficiency of certain vitamins may cause neurological injury. Vitamin deficiency may occur because of malnutrition, restricted food intake, or malabsorption. Strict vegetarian diets, for example, may be deficient in B-12, which is found primarily in animal protein; supplements may be necessary. Excessive vitamin intake also poses a risk, especially with fat-soluble vitamins, which are stored in the body. For example, excess vitamin A may cause brain

THE DECADE OF THE BRAIN

The U.S. Congress has designated the years 1990 to 2000 as the *Decade of the Brain.* The intent is both to focus public attention on neurological disorders and to recognize the tremendous advances in the understanding and treatment made possible by modern molecular biological techniques and improved management, including preventive therapy. For example, the incidence of stroke can be reduced by improved medical management of hypertension, the most common risk factor. Genetic research has led to the discovery of genes responsible for or strongly associated with several chronic degenerative diseases: muscular dystrophy, Huntington's chorea, and Alzheimer's dementia. This information is valuable for genetic counseling and will be useful for the development of therapeutic intervention, including gene therapy.

Although some neurological diseases are incurable, improved medical management and rehabilitative measures can be effective in prevention or improved survival, with a better quality of life for many patients.

swelling. Excess pyridoxine (vitamin B-6) may damage peripheral nerves.

Sexually transmitted diseases can involve the nervous system. Safer sex practices using barrier methods (condoms) are necessary to prevent damaging infections. Both syphilis and the human immunodeficiency virus (HIV), which causes AIDS, may damage the brain, spinal cord, and peripheral nerves and may be transmitted to an unborn child. For this reason, if one is sexually active and/or pregnant, and is not in a long-term, monogamous relationship, one should seek counseling and testing for sexually transmitted diseases, including AIDS.

Minimize Your Exposure to Toxic Substances

Most people require prescribed medications from time to time, and many commonly use over-the-counter drugs. The potential occurrence of side effects should not cause you to avoid necessary medications. Rather, you should have a good understanding of why you require a particular drug, as well as its potential risks and potential interactions if you are taking several drugs at one time. It is also important that you have regular medical follow-ups when taking prescription drugs. All persistent new symptoms that occur when taking a new medication should be discussed with your physician. Examples of neurological symptoms or disorders related to commonly prescribed medications include the following:

- Dizziness due to antihypertensives (may indicate excess dosage)
- Headache precipitated or exacerbated by high-estrogen birth control pills
- Involuntary movements caused by haloperidol (Haldol), an antipsychotic drug
- Peripheral neuropathy (nerve degeneration) caused by phenytoin (Dilantin), a drug commonly used to treat epilepsy.

Exposure to neurotoxins may occur in the workplace or at home. In the workplace, occupational safety regulations require explicit labeling of toxic compounds. Workplace rules that ensure safety should be followed at all times. In the home, read labels carefully and follow instructions regarding protective clothing,

WHERE VITAMINS AFFECT THE NERVOUS SYSTEM

Vitamin	Site Affected
B-1 (thiamine)	Brain, possibly peripheral nerves
B-6 (pyridoxine)	Brain, peripheral nerves
B-12	Optic nerve, brain, spinal cord, peripheral nerves
Folic Acid	Possibly peripheral nerves
Vitamin E	Eye, brain (cerebellum), peripheral nerves
B-3 (niacin)	Brain (cerebellum)
Biotin	Brain

ventilation, and disposal when using cleaning agents, paints, varnishes, artist's supplies, pesticides, or any potentially toxic substance. Known neurotoxins include carbon monoxide, methyl alcohol, benzene, carbon tetrachloride, lead, and certain pesticides.

Recreational drugs and alcohol are especially toxic to the nervous system. Regular and excessive use of alcohol can cause seizures, dementia, degeneration of the brain, and peripheral neuropathy. It may also predispose a person to certain infections. Cocaine use can result in stroke, brain hemorrhage, brain infection, and psychiatric disorders. Intravenous drug use may lead to bacterial infection of the brain and spinal cord, and is an important risk for transmission of HIV. Addiction to any of these substances is a serious medical problem with many secondary medical and social consequences. If you suspect that you have an addictive or substance abuse problem, seek medical assistance from appropriately trained personnel as soon as possible.

Think Safety

Traumatic injury to the nervous system may occur in the home, at work, or during leisure activities. To avoid potential severe damage, pay attention to safety measures and make sure that they are a part of your daily routine. Everyday safety precautions should include use of the following:

- Safety belts in automobiles
- Helmets when recommended for a sport, such as cycling or skating
- Other protective clothing when recommended, such as goggles, protective padding, and gloves.

If you have a neurological condition that impairs vision, balance, or coordination, discuss any planned physical activity with your physician.

Back pain is a common ailment, often related to lifestyle factors such as lack of exercise, obesity, poor posture, and engaging in activities or work that results in back strain. Attention to diet, maintaining proper weight, and an exercise regimen that strengthens abdominal and back muscles may reduce the risk of injury and any resulting involvement of the nervous system.

NEUROLOGICAL EVALUATION AND DIAGNOSIS

Since many apparent neurological disorders may be due to a systemic illness, consult a primary care physician first for a general evaluation and for referral to a neurologist, if appropriate.

Confirming a specific neurological disease is sometimes an arduous process, requiring the expertise of several specialists. Those who may be necessary include the following:

- Ophthalmologists (eye)
- Otolaryngologists (ear, nose, and throat)
- Neurosurgeons
- Neuroradiologists
- Psychiatrists
- Orthopedic surgeons
- Vascular surgeons
- Speech and swallowing pathologists
- Rehabilitative medicine specialists
- Medical subspecialists: rheumatology, infectious disease, cardiology, and others
- Geneticists

The growth of neurological knowledge since the 1970s is due in part to neurological subspecialists who are experts in the management of particular diseases, such as epilepsy, Parkinson's disease, muscle diseases, and multiple sclerosis. A general neurologist may be able to diagnose and treat most nervous system disorders, but difficult or atypical cases may be referred to a neurological subspecialist for management advice or continued care.

When consulting a specialist such as a neurologist, it is useful to make notes before the visit of the symptoms you wish to discuss. The sequence and timing of these symptoms or other events is important neurological information to include. The physician will ask you specific questions relating to a detailed clinical history. If mental or language impairment is present, a family member or friend should provide medical information. Medications, drug and alcohol use, and potential expo-

SPECIALISTS IN NEUROLOGICAL DISORDERS

Your primary care physician may refer you to a number of specialists who treat various aspects of diseases of the nervous system and their symptoms. Depending on the nature of the problem, they may work as a team. The team may include any or all of the following health care professionals:

- Neurologist—a doctor who specializes in the nervous system and its disorders
- Neuroradiologist—a doctor who specializes in imaging tests of the nervous system
- Neurosurgeon—a doctor who specializes in surgery of the nervous system, including the brain and the spinal cord
- Psychiatrist—a doctor who specializes in mental disorders
- Physical therapist—a trained professional who helps patients with movement disorders through manipulative exercises
- Speech therapist—a trained professional who provides guidance and therapy to overcome speech problems and to relearn speech patterns.

sures to toxic or infectious substances are important to report. Family history is important for diagnosis of genetic disorders, and even travel history may be relevant.

The preliminary physical exam will test how well the various parts of your nervous system are functioning. Tests may include your tendon reflexes, muscle strength and tone, sensory functions, and your mental state.

COMMON NEUROLOGICAL SIGNS AND SYMPTOMS

The goal of the diagnostic evaluation is to determine the cause of a specific symptom. *Symptoms* are the subjective feelings that you may experience as a patient. *Signs* are objective abnormalities detected by the physician. Symptoms such as dizziness, headache, or other pain may be disabling but not result in abnormal signs or be due to neurological injury. Other symptoms, such as loss of sensation, paralysis, or language disturbance are suggestive of neurological injury. Treatment may be directed to the underlying cause, or to amelioration of the symptom if a specific cause is not identified or cannot be treated. Sometimes, despite aggressive efforts, a cause cannot be determined.

Headache

Most people experience headaches at one time or another. In most cases, headaches are benign, temporary, and spontaneously resolved or respond to over-the-counter pain medications. In some cases, however, the symptom is incapacitating, chronic, or recurrent. Headache can also be a symptom of a serious medical condition. Age of onset and the character of the headache (quality, location, duration, and time course) are important for a specific diagnosis. Associated or precipitating factors are also useful information:

- Head trauma
- Relationship to menses
- Ingestion of hormonal active medications such as birth control pills

- Diet
- Alcohol
- Medications
- Use of illegal drugs
- Exposure to toxic substances.

The characteristics of headaches due to serious medical problems, such as a brain tumor, tend to overlap those of benign origin, such as tension or migraine. Brain tumor headaches may be mild; conversely, migraine or tension headaches may be severe. Medical evaluation is indicated for chronic headache especially if the pain is present when lying down or on arising, if the headache is of sudden onset, or if it is associated with symptoms such as fever, vomiting, behavioral change, visual disturbance, or loss of motor strength, sensation, or balance.

Your primary care physician or internist can refer you to a specialist, such as an ophthalmologist or neurologist, when necessary. A clinical history, physical examination, and baseline laboratory data such as a blood count and blood chemistry profile (including serum glucose) may be sufficient for diagnosis. Specialized diagnostic procedures may be ordered on the basis of the physician's assessment of your history and examination. These procedures may include brain imaging with computerized tomography (CT), magnetic resonance imaging (MRI), lumbar puncture, cerebral angiography, and biopsy of cerebral vessels or brain tissue. In most cases, however, these specialized tests are not required for diagnosis.

The management of primary headache disorders (migraine and tension headaches) is discussed later in this chapter. Secondary headaches due to an underlying disorder, such as hemorrhage, infection, tumor, or sinus disease, is managed by treatment of the underlying cause.

Dizziness, Vertigo, Hearing Loss

Dizziness is a nonspecific complaint that is differentiated from the more specific problem of true vertigo, although some may use these terms interchangeably. The differentiation of the nonspecific symptom of dizziness from true vertigo is based on careful history and physical examination.

Dizziness is a term used to describe diverse sensory experiences, among them giddiness, light-headedness, unsteadiness, faintness, and true vertigo. Certain types of seizures may be referred to as "dizzy spells" or may have a vertiginous component.

Vertigo is a sensation of movement of either the environment or the body. The room may seem to spin, for example, or to rotate, or move to and fro or up and down. Or you may experience a forcible pull toward the ground (impulsion). Associated symptoms usually include nausea, vomiting, imbalance, and an inability to walk. Tinnitus (a ringing or roaring sound in the ear) and hearing loss may occur. During attacks of vertigo, abnormal jerky horizontal or vertical eye movements, termed *nystagmus*, may be observed.

Normally, we maintain postural control and an awareness of the position of the body in space through a complex coordination of vision and sensory input from the eyes, ears, and specialized sensory organs (propioceptors) in the neck, muscles, and joints. These incoming sensory data are coordinated in the brain. Disturbance in any of these pathways may cause dizziness or true vertigo.

True vertigo is usually due to disturbances of the vestibular system, which includes the organs of the inner ear, the auditory nerve, and various vestibular nuclei in the brain stem. The goal of the initial evaluation of vertigo is to localize the site causing the symptom, whether it is in the labyrinth of the ear or in the central brain stem.

The labyrinth of the inner ear consists of three semicircular canals that are connected to saclike swellings, the utricle and saccule, that connect in turn to a spiral structure, the cochlea (see Fig. 2.6). These hollow canals are filled with fluid whose movement across specialized cells triggers impulses to the brain to maintain balance. Abnormalities in movement of the fluid, degeneration of the sensory receptor, and debris in the system are all potential triggers of vertigo. Often a viral inflammation is suspected.

Problems in the labyrinth may also involve mixed signals being sent from the nerve cells in the inner ear to the brain. They include a condition called Ménière's disease (see the section "Common Neurological Disorders"); positional vertigo, in which symptoms occur only when the body is in certain positions; vestibular neuronitis, acute, usually self-limiting attacks of vertigo that can follow a viral infection; and problems that are responses to certain antibiotics. Problems in the brain or its connecting nerves result when there is damage to the nerves or the brain stem and the messages are not reaching the brain. This can occur with a tumor, which can press on a nerve, or with a stroke. Other neurological diseases, such as multiple sclerosis and Parkinson's disease, can involve damage to the sensory nerves, which can result in dizziness as well as a number of other symptoms.

Certain drugs—among them salicylates (aspirin-containing compounds), quinine, and aminoglycoside antibiotics—may cause tinnitus, hearing loss, and vertigo. Nonvertiginous dizziness has many causes and requires a detailed history and examination to determine the cause. Most often, the cause is nonneurological—for example, severe anemia, low blood sugar, drug side effects, low blood pressure, or high blood pressure. Your primary care physician will seek to exclude these causes during the medical evaluation.

Diagnostic tests to investigate true vertigo include an audiogram, to test hearing; calorics, which involve irrigation of the ears with hot and cold water, to assess labyrinthine and brain stem function; electronystagmography, a test to detect abnormal eye movements (nystagmus); and tests to assess nerve and brain stem function. If imaging is necessary, an MRI with contrast is the procedure of choice.

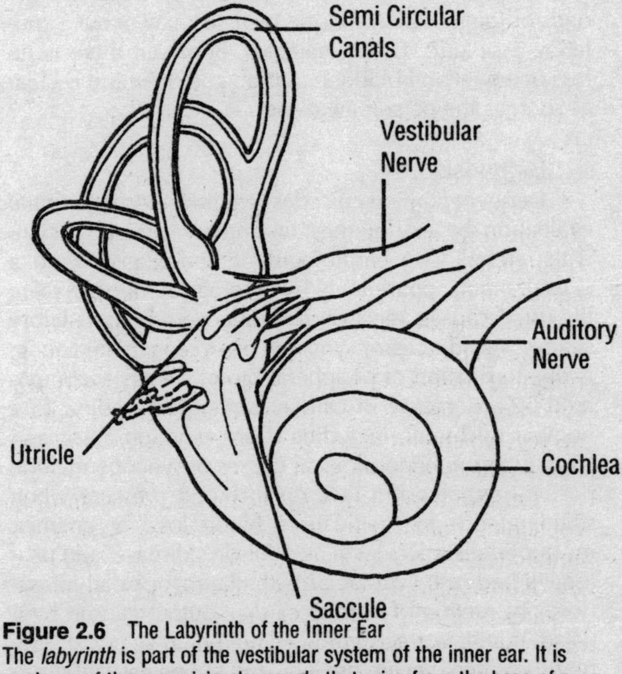

Figure 2.6 The Labyrinth of the Inner Ear
The *labyrinth* is part of the vestibular system of the inner ear. It is made up of three semicircular canals that arise from the base of a rounded chamber called the vestibule. Within the vestibule are two fluid-filled sacs called the utricle and the saccule, which are connected to the cochlea.

Fainting, or Syncope

Syncope is a medical term referring to loss of consciousness and postural control, commonly called a *faint.* Prodromal (warning) symptoms usually occur, including light-headedness or giddiness, dim vision, and stomach discomfort or queasiness. Lying down may abort the attack. Although there is usually complete loss of contact with the environment during syncope, in some cases the person is vaguely aware of what is going on around her or him. With prolonged syncope (20 seconds or longer), brief muscle twitches may occur, simulating a seizure. Unlike seizures, however, there is no loss of bowel and bladder control, and the mind is clear as soon as the person awakens.

Diagnosis

Frequent fainting episodes require a thorough initial evaluation by an internist or primary care physician, with referral to a cardiologist or neurologist when a cause is not apparent. Nonneurological disorders are the usual causes, most of them affecting the circulatory system. Vasodepressor syncope, often seen in the young, is due to dilation of peripheral blood vessels accompanied by a decrease in cardiac output in response to a number of stimuli, including strong emotion, heat, and pain. Other nonneurological causes of syncope include postural hypotension (a drop in blood pressure when standing) due to medication, blood loss, or anemia; metabolic disorders such as Addison's disease; and prolonged bed rest. Cardiac arrhythmia, myocardial infarction, obstruction of normal cardiac output caused by a narrow outflow tract (aortic or pulmonic stenosis), low blood oxygen, severe anxiety, and hyperventilation are other causes. Unusual occurrences of syncope are following urination (micturition syncope), after a paroxysm of coughing (tussive syncope), and after eating (postprandial syncope). Abnormal slowing of the heart rate by excessive discharge of the vagus nerve (one of the nerves to the heart) is the suspected cause.

A neurologist is involved in the evaluation of syncope because neurological conditions may cause a fainting fit and seizure disorder must be excluded.

Syncope may occur in the context of stroke but is rarely the sole symptom. Distinguishing syncope from seizure is often difficult and requires taking a careful history. An electroencephalogram (EEG) is sometimes helpful, although a normal study will not entirely exclude seizures.

Sometimes, despite extensive investigations, a cause for syncope is not determined. In this case, regular follow-up is advisable, with repeat diagnostic testing as events warrant. In some cases psychiatric referral is necessary because panic attacks, anxiety, and other psychiatric problems may cause syncope or apparent syncope.

Treatment

The prevention and treatment of syncope depends on the cause. Interventions include a change in medication, fluid or blood replacement, and glucose control. In hyperventilation, breathing into a paper bag prevents the extreme loss of carbon dioxide that causes dizziness and syncope. Measures useful for treatment of neurogenic low blood pressure are elevation of the head of the bed when sleeping; elastic stockings and abdominal binders to increase blood return to the heart; increased salt intake; and medications such as fludrocortisone acetate (Florinef), tyramine, monoamine oxidase inhibitors, beta-blockers, and indomethacin.

Pain

Neurological evaluation is often necessary for persons suffering from acute or chronic pain syndromes. Physicians who may be involved in pain assessment and care include internists or primary care physicians, orthopedic surgeons, neurosurgeons, physiatrists (rehabilitation medicine specialists), psychiatrists, and anesthesiologists. The neurologist is specifically concerned with pain in the head, neck, back, and limbs. In some cases of chronic pain, a multidisciplinary team of several specialists provides care.

Acute, Persistent Pain

Severe pain in the structures of the nervous system requires prompt evaluation. Consult your primary care physician to determine the appropriate referral. For some acute pain syndromes, however, immediate help may be needed. You may require an emergency room evaluation, especially if you have no primary physician or if the associated symptoms or signs suggest an emergency condition. Emergency conditions include brain or spine hemorrhage or infection, and pressure on the brain or spine due to tumor or other causes. In these conditions, pain is of sudden onset or builds in intensity over a few days. Associated signs or symptoms that may indicate an emergency situation are fever and change in mental function, strength, sensation, or gait. In spine compression, difficulty urinating may occur.

Assessment of acute pain always begins with a detailed history and examination. In emergency conditions, treatment may be initiated before diagnostic tests are ordered. The doctor will ensure that all the vital organs are functioning properly. In some cases, a tube will be inserted into the trachea and a respirator used to support ventilation. This technique is especially useful if there is brain swelling or mental function is depressed.

A catheter may be inserted to drain the bladder and monitor urine output. Intravenous fluids may be given. Pain medications are sometimes withheld until the diagnosis is secure because mental function may need to be followed. If there is pressure on the brain or spine, steroids or mannitol may be given to reduce swelling. Studies that may be necessary include MRI, CT, angiography, and myelography. Whenever infection is suspected, lumbar puncture must be done without delay for diagnosis unless there is suspicion of a mass lesion, such as an abscess. Lumbar puncture is also useful for diagnosis of brain hemorrhage.

Emergency conditions may require the patient or the family to make decisions about procedures or surgery in the space of a few hours. It is important to recognize that when a neurological emergency exists, delays in treatment may cause irreversible injury or death.

Chronic Pain Syndromes

Intermittent, chronic pain requires multidisciplinary management. Important information for a correct diagnosis includes the location of pain and its radiation, character, and duration. Also important is your response to medications or different postures, and any association of the pain with neurological abnormalities such as change in mental function, sensation, strength, or gait. A prior history of trauma or medical conditions such as diabetes, cancer, or infections (Lyme disease, HIV, *Herpes zoster*) is also relevant. In some cases, history and examination are sufficient for diagnosis; in others, diagnostic tests are necessary, including imaging studies, lumbar puncture, and electromyography (EMG), a test of nerve function.

As stated previously, headache is the commonest cause of head pain. There are other pain syndromes called neuralgias, pains in a specific nerve pattern in the head. Sometimes the pain is caused by inflammation of the brain or blood vessels in the head, as in cranial arteritis. Temporomandibular joint (TMJ) problems may cause head pain and are diagnosed by examination and X-ray.

Trigeminal Neuralgia

Also known as tic douloureux, *trigeminal neuralgia* occurs in middle age and later life, and is characterized by repetitive bursts of severe pain in the face, most often in the cheek. The pain is in the distribution of the fifth cranial nerve (trigeminal nerve), which has three branches: the first to the eye area (ophthalmic), the second to the cheek and nose area (mandibular), and the third to the lower face and chin (maxillary). Facial weakness and sensory loss do not usually occur. The pain is often triggered by stimulation to the face, mouth, and gums, as occurs in shaving, brushing the teeth, yawning, or chewing. Exposure to air may also precipitate episodes of pain. Attacks often occur in clusters that last for days, weeks, or months, followed by spontaneous remission.

A symptomatic tic may be due to a tumor, dental problems, multiple sclerosis, or an aneurysm; the cause is determined by examination and imaging studies, usually MRI. Sometimes the tic is caused by a blood vessel pressing on the nerve.

Several medications are useful for pain control, including antiepileptic drugs such as phenytoin (Dilantin) and carbamazepine (Tegretol); the tricyclic antidepressant amitriptyline (Elavil); clonazepam (Klonopin); and baclofen (Lioresal). Sometimes drugs are combined when a single drug is insufficient for pain control. Surgery is available for those with intractable pain. The traditional method of treatment involved injection of alcohol or phenol into the nerve root, resulting in loss of facial sensation. Two surgical methods currently used are the Janetta procedure, a technique of nerve decompression when pain is due to pressure by a blood vessel, and stereotactic radio-frequency thermocoagulation, a technique that heats the nerve. The Janetta procedure does not cause sensory loss.

Temporal Arteritis

This condition is a cause of headache in the older population, age of onset usually in the mid-50s, and is less common in women. Pain is caused by inflammation of the blood vessels. Diagnosis is by biopsy of the temporal artery, an uncomplicated office procedure. If it is not diagnosed, blindness may occur because of involvement of ophthalmic blood vessels. Involvement of large vessels in the brain can cause a stroke. Steroids are an effective treatment.

Herpes Zoster Infection (Shingles)

Shingles may involve the face and other parts of the body. This viral infection responds to treatment with acyclovir (Zovirax) or is self-limited. Some people, particularly women, develop a severe pain syndrome in the affected area that is called postherpetic neuralgia. In most cases the pain resolves after two to three months. In others, however, the pain may become chronic and intractable. Medical management is similar to that for tic douloureux, with amitriptyline (Elavil) the preferred drug. Phenothiazine medications are also useful but may have unacceptable side effects. Topical treatment with capsaicin (a counterirritant) or the use of local anesthetic sprays and a technique called transcutaneous electrical stimulation (TENS) may benefit some shingles sufferers.

Back Pain

One of the most common ailments, back pain affects up to 20 percent of the U.S. population. It is the commonest cause of disability in people under age 45, with 6 to 8 million persons claiming disability for this problem.

Many women are at special risk because of sedentary lifestyles, pregnancy, household and child care activities, and postmenopausal thinning of bone (osteoporosis). Maintaining proper weight, regular exercise, and good nutrition with adequate intake of vitamin D and calcium reduce the risk of back problems. Because household chores and child care involve repetitive lifting, bending, and stooping, it pays to learn proper lifting techniques. In postmenopausal women, estrogen replacement therapy may lessen the severity of osteoporosis. (See Part III)

In the evaluation of a patient with neck or lower back pain, the neurologist first determines if there is injury to the spinal cord or nerves. This may be obvious if there is weakness or loss of muscle tissue. Conversely, the damage may be detectable only by examination, which consists of inspection and palpation of the spine and joints; observation of gait; tests of spine mobility; attempts to elicit pain by palpation, punch, and spine or limb movement; tests of sensory perception by light touch, pinprick, application of heat and cold, and vibration; and tests of individual muscle strength and reflexes.

Severe back pain may also result from spasm of neck or back muscles. Strains or sprains can be caused by whiplash injury, heavy lifting, or twisting injury to the spine, even without structural injury to the spinal cord or nerves. Such pain results from the stretching or tearing of support structures such as ligaments and tendons. Pain that radiates down a limb in a localized distribution, called radiculopathy, suggests pressure on a nerve or root. Sciatica, pain radiating from the hip down the back of the leg, is an example. Pressure on the spinal cord causes pain over the affected area and may result in leg weakness, walking problems, or urinary incontinence.

Diagnosis

Diagnostic tests include X-rays, imaging studies (CT, MRI, myelography), and EMG. The extent and promptness of the testing depend on the history and examination, not just the severity of pain.

The purpose of the diagnostic tests is to identify a structural cause for the pain, such as disc bulge, tumor, infection, or arthritis. It is important to recognize, however, that structural abnormalities such as disc bulges and arthritis are common in adults and may not be responsible for the pain in question.

Treatment

Pain due to structural spine problems may be managed conservatively with rest, pain medication, and a supervised therapy program, or may require surgery. Both orthopedic surgeons and neurosurgeons evaluate and operate on spine problems. If surgery is recommended, make sure you obtain more than one opinion, especially if the problem identified is arthritis or disc disease. If the spinal cord is compressed by a tumor, disc, or abscess, emergency surgery may be necessary to prevent irreversible paralysis and incontinence.

Most lower back pain is not due to structural spine disease. Lax ligaments, poor muscle tone, poor posture, and obesity are contributing factors. Psychological problems can also contribute to the severity and chronicity of the pain. Weight reduction and regular exercise are appropriate nonsurgical treatment of pain. Stress management, biofeedback, and acupuncture are also sometimes recommended. Nonnarcotic analgesics may be used for pain relief; amitriptyline benefits some.

Narcotic drugs should be reserved for those with cancer and with severe pain.

Myofascial Pain Syndrome

This refers to localized areas of muscle pain and tenderness called "trigger points." It may exist with other pain syndromes, and the cause is uncertain. Prior trauma, such as whiplash injury, plays a role in some cases. The diagnosis is by clinical examination. Treatment consists of massage; acupressure; acupuncture; local application of heat, cold, or topical sprays; and an exercise regimen. Trigger point injections of local anesthetics and steroids are also helpful. Stress reduction and regular exercise prevent relapse.

Stupor and Coma

Stupor is an altered state of consciousness in which a person appears sleepy or lethargic but can be roused. *Coma* is a state of unconsciousness from which a person cannot be roused. Any abrupt change in mental state or level of consciousness requires prompt evaluation in an emergency room. Emergency transport personnel will assess the vital signs and administer appropriate treatment en route to the hospital. If breathing is compromised, a tube will be inserted into the trachea for delivery of oxygen. Narcan (a drug to reverse drug overdose), glucose, thiamine, and intravenous fluids are usually given. In trauma cases, the spine is immobilized in case there is unrecognized injury.

Once the patient is in the hospital, medical specialists and neurologists will determine if the coma is due to a systemic problem (drug overdose, diabetes, low blood sugar, exposure to a toxic substance) or a primary neurological event (meningitis, encephalitis, brain hemorrhage, or stroke). Recovery from coma is dependent on cause and duration. In prolonged coma, care includes nutritional support and prevention of pneumonia, skin breakdown and blood clots in the legs and lungs. Some causes of coma result in brain death. This diagnosis is determined by both clinical and electrical (EEG) criteria. (Most medical institutions have a protocol for determination of brain death.) Clinical criteria include no evidence of speech or comprehension; no volitional movement or response to pain; no spontaneous respiration; no eye movements or pupil reflexes; no limb reflexes. The examination is repeated after several hours to determine irreversibility. The EEG is flat, indicating no cerebral activity.

Brain death cannot be diagnosed immediately after cardiac arrest or in the presence of severe hypothermia or high levels of sedative/hypnotic drugs. A person may meet all criteria for brain death and still show reflex leg or toe movements due to spinal reflexes.

In cases of coma with partial recovery, a persistent vegetative state may ensue. The person may exhibit spontaneous blinking, roving eye movements, and reflex limb movements in response to touch or pain, but no pattern can be established.

COMMON NEUROLOGICAL DISORDERS

Neurological disorders can be self-limiting (disappear on their own) or have symptoms that come and go over a long period. Sometimes the symptoms become progressively worse. In many cases, treatment is available to control symptoms and prevent progression of the disease.

Migraine Headache

Migraine headaches are common in the U.S. population, affecting 7.4 percent of women and 3.5 percent of men. The first attack is most often in the late teens or in young adulthood but may occur at any age. Childhood onset is not uncommon. In some women, the headaches occur in the premenstrual period. Fifty to 70 percent of cases are familial, indicating an inherited disorder.

Migraine is a recurrent, throbbing headache accompanied by complex symptoms suggesting a systemic disorder. In most sufferers, there are at least three distinct phases: the prodrome (symptoms that precede the headache), the headache phase, and the post-headache period. The symptom complex may last several days. The prodrome consists of an altered psychic state that may be reflected in sudden, increased energy a few days preceding the headache. Headache may then begin suddenly or build slowly after an *aura* or brief warning.

The aura may be visual, sensory, psychic, or motor, and usually lasts 10 to 20 minutes before onset of the headache. Visual auras, the most common, consist of zigzag lines, flashes of white or colored light, or other distortions that move across the visual field, leaving a blind spot or an inability to see to one side. Sensory symptoms consist of numbness and tingling of lips or limbs. Disturbances of mood, mental confusion, and language problems may also occur.

A migraine headache is classified as common, classic, or complicated. *Common migraine* is a headache without aura. It occurs in almost 90 percent of migraine sufferers. *Classic migraine* is migraine with an aura. There are other specific migraine patterns with associated neurological symptoms or signs, such as unilateral dilated pupil, droopy lid, and paralysis of eye movement (ophthalmoplegic migraine), vertigo and imbalance (basilar migraine), and unilateral limb paralysis (hemiplegic migraine). These types of migraine headaches are usually hereditary and often begin in childhood.

The migraine headache is usually very severe, often beginning in a localized area, such as above or behind the eye, then spreading to half the head before becoming generalized. Nausea and vomiting occur with both common and classic migraine. Sensitivity to light and sound is usual, and skin color and temperature changes sometimes occur. Most sufferers seek rest in a quiet, darkened environment. Once the headache has abated, fatigue and drowsiness are common complaints.

Diagnosis

The diagnosis of migraine is based on history and examination. If the neurological examination is normal, the diagnostic evaluation may be limited to examination and baseline blood studies. Diagnostic tests such as brain imaging with MRI or CT and angiography are indicated in older persons and those with complicated migraine. Lumbar puncture may be indicated because the migraine headache may mimic the headache of brain hemorrhage or infection.

Treatment

The management of migraine has three objectives: aborting the attack, pain relief, and prevention of further episodes. Migraine aura and other neurological symptoms are due to constriction of blood vessels in the brain; the pain is caused by excessive blood vessel dilation. Medications that abort headache prevent excess vasodilation.

Two drugs specifically abort headache: ergotamine tartrate derivatives and sumatriptin (Imitrex). One derivative, Cafergot, is a combination of ergotamine and caffeine. Ergotamine derivatives are available in tablets for oral or sublingual use, rectal suppositories and injectable solutions. Imitrex is available for injection only and comes in a preloaded kit for self-administration. Your physician can provide training in self-injection techniques. A medication given by injection or a rectal suppository is preferred because tablets may not be well absorbed. The dosage of ergotamine derivative and Imitrex is limited because of serious side effects from overuse. Pregnant women and those with complicated migraine should not use these vasoconstrictive medications.

A number of other medications are available for pain relief, and some of them are also effective in aborting attacks. Your physician will outline the types you may try, ranging from over-the-counter medications such as aspirin, acetaminophen (Tylenol), and nonsteroidal drugs like ibuprofen (Advil, Motrin) to prescription drugs. Avoid those with addictive potential, especially narcotics, unless they are absolutely necessary for pain control. Finding the appropriate medication is a trial-and-error process. Medication overdosage can worsen the headache. If you suffer from migraine and take several analgesic tablets daily, yet experience daily morning headache, you are likely suffering from medication overdosage.

Preventive therapy is necessary in cases of frequent migraine. Stress management, regular exercise, dietary changes, and biofeedback are beneficial. Possible food triggers for migraine include chocolate, nuts, aged cheese, citrus fruits, bananas, monosodium glutamate (present in some Chinese food and used as a flavor enhancer), dairy products, pickles, cured meats, and alcohol. Birth control pills and the antihypertensive drug reserpine may trigger or cause migraine.

Prophylactic drugs are usually given until a painfree state is achieved for several months. Medication may then be tapered off and discontinued. Abrupt discontinuation of medication may provoke severe rebound migraine or *status migrainosus,* a syndrome of almost continuous headache that requires hospital management. Prophylactic medications for migraine include beta-blockers such as propranolol (Inderal); calcium channel blockers (verapamil, nifedipine); methysergide (Sansert), a long-acting ergot derivative; and amitriptyline (Elavil). Indomethacin (Indocin) is often useful in premenstrual migraine.

Cluster headache is a variant of migraine that usually affects adult men. This type of headache is among the worst, typically awakening the sufferer from sleep. Unlike migraine sufferers, those with cluster headaches are unable to rest and are agitated and restless, sometimes in such great pain that suicide is contemplated. *Tension headache* is regarded as a musculoskeletal contraction headache, with pain usually described as squeezing or viselike. Its characteristics may overlap those of migraine, and it may be as severe as, or coexist with, typical migraine.

Spine and Disc Disorders

Degenerative changes in the spine are an inevitable part of aging. Bone, ligaments, tendons, and the intervertebral discs are affected. The lower part of the neck and lower back are at greatest risk for degenerative change. Osteoporosis or multiple pregnancies in women are aggravating factors.

Osteoporosis causes thinning of bone that may result in painful vertebral collapse. Immobilization is the usual treatment, with gradual return to movement in a supervised therapy program. A cervical collar or a lower back support brace is prescribed.

Arthritic spine changes result in bony overgrowth that narrows the spinal canal, causing spinal stenosis.

Pain in the legs when walking is a symptom of spinal stenosis. Pain is treated with bed rest, analgesics, cervical collar or back brace, and physical therapy. Prolonged use of a back brace is usually not recommended because it weakens abdominal muscles. Surgery is indicated for intractable, severe pain and for those with signs of nerve or spinal cord injury.

Disc disease may be due to degeneration of the disc itself or to degeneration of the ligaments that hold the disc in place. Disc herniation is extrusion of the disc into the spinal canal, where it may compress a nerve or the spinal cord. Disc disease and arthritis can exist together.

The nature and extent of surgical intervention depend on the spine problem. For spinal stenosis or disc degeneration and spinal stenosis, more extensive surgical procedures may be necessary to relieve pressure on the spine and nerve roots.

Sometimes surgery fails to relieve pain. This may not be due to a failure in surgical technique but to factors beyond the surgeon's control, such as postoperative scarring or a persistent, inflammatory reaction at the operated site (arachnoiditis). Persistent or recurrent postoperative pain requires reevaluation with imaging studies. If no new surgical problem is identified, long-term physical therapy is indicated.

Head and Brain Injury

Traumatic head injury requires prompt medical evaluation because of the potential for serious brain damage. Head injury may result from blunt trauma due to a blow or fall, indirect trauma such as blast injury or whiplash, or penetrating trauma, as with a bullet wound.

Head injury with skull fracture and penetrating head wounds have the highest potential for significant brain injury. There may be hemorrhage into brain tissue or between the membranes overlying the brain (subdural or epidural hematoma). Loss of consciousness usually occurs with significant brain injury, but in some cases is brief. This brief unconsciousness in an apparently lucid person may mask serious injury, however, and is characteristic of epidural hematomas that then suddenly enlarge, causing severe brain compression and death if untreated.

Concussion refers to the loss of consciousness after a head injury. *Contusion* refers to a brain injury similar to a bruise. After concussion, a person may show no symptoms or may experience symptoms of amnesia in regard to the injury and the immediate surrounding time period, dizziness, tinnitus, and headache. In some cases, mood changes, irritability, loss of interest in usual activities, slowed thinking, poor concentration, and depression may occur. The symptoms may last several weeks or months. This postconcussion syndrome is sometimes seen with even minor head injuries. Antidepressants may be beneficial for control of headache and depression. Neurological signs may occur with severe cerebral contusion, resulting in slow or incomplete recovery.

Complications of head injury include meningitis and brain abscess. Impact seizures occur at the time of injury and do not predict a future seizure disorder. Permanent seizure disorders are more likely with penetrating wounds. Seizures that occur more than a month after injury are called posttraumatic epilepsy.

Victims of significant head trauma are assessed and stabilized medically to ensure that other vital structures are not injured. Medications to prevent seizures and treat brain swelling are given. The neck should be immobilized until X-rays are taken because neck injury can escape detection in the unconscious head-injured person. Imaging studies, usually CT, are obtained. If a large hematoma is visualized, emergency drainage is performed. Small hematomas may be followed by means of periodic examination and scans. In some penetrating injuries, such as bullet wounds, surgery may be limited to removing dead tissue and cleansing the area, because removal of the bullet or its fragments is too risky.

Recovery after head injury may be gradual and prolonged if neurologic deficits are severe. Cognitive remedial therapy is important for those with memory and language deficits.

Epilepsy

A seizure is a behavioral or neurological event caused by abnormal electrical discharge in the brain. Recurrent seizures are called epilepsy. The behaviors observed before and during a seizure include staring spells with inattention, repetitive automatic movements or gestures, repetitive jerks of a limb, and loss of consciousness with generalized jerking of the limbs and back arching. Tongue biting and urinary incontinence can occur. Confusion, amnesia, and agitation can follow a generalized seizure.

Diagnosis

Persons with possible seizures should be evaluated by an experienced primary care clinician, internist, or neurologist. The primary care physician or internist will look for toxic or metabolic causes of seizures. The neurologist will look for neurological abnormalities that could indicate a brain lesion. The history is the most important part of the diagnostic evaluation. Family history, birth injury, head trauma, and infection, among others, are important in determining if a single seizure will lead to epilepsy. Some seizure disorders are inherited.

Diagnostic tests include baseline blood tests (blood

count, serum glucose, and chemistry profile), EEG, and brain imaging. Lumbar puncture is sometimes recommended. You may be asked to remain awake the night before an EEG and be given a mild sedative during the test. This is done to "activate" abnormal electrical discharges. During the test other activators, such as flashing lights and rapid breathing, are used. Without activation, an EEG is likely to be normal between seizures. Sometimes it is normal despite their use. Repeat studies are sometimes done, and in some cases video-EEG is performed. Video-EEG is done in a hospital setting with continuous EEG and camera monitoring for 24–48 hours. This is useful for determining if an event is a seizure and for localizing the seizure discharge.

The results of the history, examination, and diagnostic tests are used to classify epilepsy as partial, primary, or symptomatic. *Partial* seizures originate in a localized area of the brain but may spread to the whole brain, becoming secondarily generalized. Temporal lobe and complex partial seizures are examples of partial seizures. Seizures may also be diagnosed as *primary,* not associated with a brain lesion, or *symptomatic,* due to a brain lesion such as tumor, stroke, vascular malformation, trauma, or birth injury.

Treatment

The classification of the seizures determines the selection of the most effective drug therapy. There are several medications for treatment of epilepsy, but single drug therapy is preferred. If the initial drug selected does not work, the neurologist will substitute another, rather than prescribe a combination of two. In difficult cases, multiple drugs may be necessary. Blood levels are monitored to ensure adequate dosage. Anticonvulsant medication may have side effects, so medical follow-up is necessary.

Symptomatic seizures may require treatment of the

precipitating cause as well as medication for the seizures. Chronic alcoholism, for example, may lead to a seizure disorder that occurs only during periods of abstinence. Drug use and dependence may also cause seizures. These seizures usually remit with abstinence. Medication is not necessary unless there is a coexistent brain injury.

Surgery is performed for severe epilepsy that does not respond to medical management. Such surgery is available in specialized centers and requires careful evaluation, including brain mapping, to isolate the focus of the seizure discharge. Success rates may approach 50 percent with a cure or improved response to medication.

Persons with epilepsy who are neurologically normal and whose seizures are well controlled may live a normal life and participate in all activities. Some jobs and activities may pose a risk if there are occasional breakthrough seizures. Appropriate activities should be discussed with the doctor. Driving is not restricted if seizures are controlled. State laws should be checked for requirements of reporting and medical clearance.

If seizures are controlled for several years, your physician may recommend gradual discontinuation of medication. The physician will consider several factors, including the seizure type and EEG findings. Never make this decision on your own without medical supervision. Abrupt discontinuation of seizure medication may cause *status epilepticus,* frequently recurring seizures with unconsciousness, a neurological emergency.

Strokes

Stroke is one of the most common disorders of the nervous system. The term is often used interchangeably with *cerebrovascular accident* (CVA), implying a vascular cause. Because not all neurological impairments that resemble a stroke are of vascular origin, the term *stroke syndrome* is preferred. Diagnostic tests are necessary to determine if a vascular event is the cause.

A stroke is a focal neurological abnormality that occurs suddenly or over a period of a few hours. Strokelike symptoms that are transient and fully resolvable, lasting from minutes up to 24 hours, are called *transient ischemic attacks* (TIAs).

Vascular stroke is caused by hemorrhage in the brain or blockage of a blood vessel by a clot (embolus or thrombus). The neurological deficit occurs because a portion of the brain is deprived of oxygen or compressed by the bleeding. Bleeding into the brain may be caused by trauma, bleeding disorders like hemophilia, tumor, a ruptured aneurysm, vascular malformation, cocaine use, hypertension, a degenerative blood vessel disease, or amyloid. Inflammation of blood vessels (vasculitis) may also lead to hemorrhage or infarct. Stroke due to blockage of a vessel by clot is called cerebral infarction. A thrombus may form in a blood vessel narrowed by atherosclerosis or damaged by hypertension. The heart may be a source of an embolus, a clot that travels to a blood vessel from a distant site. Embolic infarctions may be associated with bleeding. Abnormal heart valves, irregular heart rhythms, and myocardial infarction may all lead to stroke. Conversely, those who have stroke are at significant risk for coronary artery disease.

The symptoms and signs of stroke depend on the area of the brain affected. There may be visual problems such as blindness in one eye, double vision, or inability to see to one side; difficulty understanding or speaking; weakness of an arm and leg; or unsteadiness when walking.

Diagnosis

Imaging studies such as CT or MRI determine the area of the brain that is affected and detect hemorrhage or other conditions, such as a tumor. Lumbar puncture is sometimes necessary. Angiography is used to identify the site of blockage as well as potential surgical problems such as aneurysm, vascular malformation, or narrowed carotid arteries. Other diagnostic tests will depend on the nature of the stroke and may include an echocardiogram to reveal abnormal heart valves or thrombus, an EKG or a 24-hour heart monitor to detect abnormal heart rhythms, an ultrasound of the large neck vessels (Doppler study), and an EEG. In some cases, special blood tests are done to detect inflammatory problems such as lupus or blood abnormalities that are associated with a clotting tendency.

Treatment

Treatment of stroke begins with prevention, which includes control of blood pressure, reduction of serum cholesterol, management of diabetes mellitus, and cessation of smoking or illicit drug use. Aspirin therapy and anticoagulants (blood thinners) are prescribed preventively to those at risk for stroke, and therapeutically to those who have suffered stroke. Surgery on the carotid artery is performed for severe blockage in those who have TIAs or minor stroke due to the blockage, or for bleeding aneurysms. Surgery is not done if the vessel is completely closed.

Following stroke, rehabilitation should begin as soon as possible. For major deficits, inpatient treatment is necessary. For those with minor disability, home-based or outpatient treatment is sufficient.

Ménière's Disease

The classic labyrinthine form of vertigo, Ménière's disease, usually occurs in the 50s; women and men are equally affected. The attacks of vertigo are abrupt and usually associated with tinnitus, diminished hearing, or a sense of fullness in the ear. Nausea, vomiting, imbalance, or an inability to walk may also occur. Rarely, the attacks are so violent that they result in sudden falls. The medical examination may disclose hearing loss, usually in one ear and generally before the first attack of vertigo, and nystagmus. The clinical course is recurrent attacks and progressive hearing loss, although the severity of the attacks lessens as hearing loss increases. In 10 percent of cases, the hearing loss is in both ears. Rarely, the disease is inherited.

Diagnosis

Although the cause of Ménière's disease is uncertain, pathologic studies often show an abnormal collection of fluid in the affected ear. It is reasonable to suggest that vertigo is precipitated by membrane rupture and the release of the fluid into the space around the nerves, resulting in damage to the vestibular nerve and cochlear cells.

Treatment

This condition is treated by bed rest and antihistamine-type medications such as dimenhydrinate (Dramamine), cyclizine (Marezine), and meclizine (Antivert). Medication for nausea and anxiety may also be prescribed. Dietary salt restriction and diuretics are sometimes recommended but are of unproven benefit. Continuous disabling vertigo may be corrected by surgical labyrinthine destruction, a treatment of last resort for those with unilateral disease. This type of surgery causes deafness.

There are other types of labyrinthine vertigo.

- *Benign positional vertigo.* A rapid change in position can cause a vertigo that can be reproduced by similar maneuvers during examination. Hearing is normal. This disorder is attributed to the dislocation of small stonelike structures (otoliths) into one of the semicircular canals. Some specialists recommend trying to displace the otoliths by lying first on the side that causes vertigo for 30 seconds, then changing to the other side. Repeat this maneuver 5 times, several times a day.

- *Vestibular neuronitis.* This benign form of vertigo often follows an infection and is usually self-limited. Vertigo may, however, be severe and sometimes recurrent.
- *Labyrinthine apoplexy.* This term applies to a syndrome of sudden vertigo with resulting destruction of the labyrinth of the inner ear. The cause is unknown.

Vertigo of vestibular nerve origin may be due to a tumor, inflammation, infection, or compression of the nerve by an adjacent artery. The most common cause is a tumor known as an acoustic neuroma. Deafness usually precedes the vertigo, and other signs may be present. Vertigo of brain stem origin is usually accompanied by other signs and symptoms. Causes include stroke, multiple sclerosis, infection, and migraine.

Parkinson's Disease

Parkinson's disease is a degenerative disease of the elderly, with peak age at onset in the 60s, although some cases are identified in persons as young as 30. The prevalence increases with advancing age. Approximately 500,000 persons in the United States have Parkinson's. The disease is rarely familial.

Parkinson's is a disorder of movement. The main features are rigidity, tremor while resting, motor slowness, postural instability, and abnormal gait. Tremor may affect hands and legs; it is worse at rest and decreases with motion. Depression and dementia may coexist, their frequency increasing with disease duration in up to half of patients.

Diagnosis

Parkinson's disease is diagnosed by a medical history and examination. The onset of the disease is sometimes so gradual that symptoms are attributed to depression or "normal" aging. Diagnostic tests are used to exclude other disorders that cause Parkinsonian symptoms (symptomatic Parkinson's). These include hydrocephalus (enlargement of the water-filled brain spaces), stroke, and other brain lesions. CT or MRI imaging is usually done to exclude these causes. Some drugs also cause a Parkinsonian state, especially the phenothiazines.

Treatment

Because Parkinson's is due to a loss of the brain chemical dopamine, drugs used to treat Parkinson's replace this chemical or act to balance the ratio between dopamine and another brain chemical, acetylcholine. There are several useful drugs: a combination of levodopa and carbidopa (Sinemet), which lessens the risk of nausea caused by levodopa alone; bromocriptine (Parlodel); a drug that acts like dopamine; seligiline (Eldepryl), a drug that may slow the progression of Parkinson's; trihexiphenidyl (Artane), a drug that lowers the level of acetylcholine; and amantidine (Symmetrel), a drug that releases dopamine from cells. Vitamin E also has been recommended to slow disease progression but is of uncertain benefit.

The management of Parkinson's disease is complex and should be done by a physician experienced in use of the available drugs. Drug combinations may be required, and sometimes a "drug holiday," when all drugs are stopped, may be necessary. Overuse of drugs can accelerate the progression of the disease or lead to unacceptable side effects, such as low blood pressure, confusion, hallucinations, and abnormal movements. Depression improves with antidepressive medication and sometimes with electroconvulsive therapy (ECT). Physical therapy is also an important part of treatment. Dietary restriction of foods containing the chemical phenylalanine may be necessary.

Multiple Sclerosis

This is the most common neurological disorder of young adults, affecting 250,000 to 350,000 people in the United States. Two-thirds of those affected have a first attack between the ages of 20 and 40. The disease occurs rarely in childhood or as late as the 50s and 60s. Women are affected two to three times more often than men, and 15 percent of cases have an affected relative.

The cause of multiple sclerosis (MS) is unknown. Factors thought to play a role are viral infectious agents, genetics, and geographic location. The incidence of the disease is much lower in equatorial regions of the world and increases at more northern latitudes. An abnormal immune response that destroys the central nervous system substance myelin (the covering of nerve fibers) is thought to trigger attacks. Although many have suggested that a virus induces the autoimmunity, no consistent relationship between a particular virus and MS has been established. Some have suggested that initial attacks or relapses are triggered by infection, trauma, or pregnancy, but others question the association of these otherwise common events with MS.

The symptoms of MS depend on the area of brain affected. Visual loss due to optic neuritis (inflammation of the optic nerve) is a common initial complaint. Up to half of persons with this problem will develop MS within 5 years. Other symptoms include double vision, slurred speech, leg stiffness, incoordination, and limb numbness, tingling, or weakness. Bladder, bowel, and sexual functions may be affected. Paroxysmal pain syndromes such as tic douloureux sometimes occur.

MS is an episodic disorder, meaning that symptoms begin abruptly and remit over several weeks. Chronic progressive MS, a less common presentation, is characterized by progressive disability without remissions. Some patients enjoy a benign course with few or nondisabling attacks, and some are asymptomatic for life, diagnosed with MS only incidentally at autopsy.

Diagnosis

Diagnosis is by clinical criteria based on neurological examination or by a combination of clinical and laboratory tests. Diagnostic tests include lumbar puncture, MRI scans of brain and/or spinal cord, and evoked potential studies. Lumbar puncture is done to test for olioclonal bands, an abnormal protein pattern found in MS but not limited to this disease. MRI identifies the white matter plaques of MS. Other tests show delay in nerve transmission caused by the loss of myelin.

Treatment

Intravenous or oral steroids can shorten acute attacks and speed recovery. Intravenous steroids are preferred for optic neuritis. Other immunosuppressive drugs sometimes given are azathioprine (Imuran) and cyclophosphamide (Cytoxan). The new drug Beta-Seron, a type of interferon, decreases the number of attacks in those who relapse. Baclofen (Lioresal) is used for spasticity. It may be given orally or intrathecally into the spinal space. Paroxysmal pain of MS may be treated with amitriptyline or other drugs.

Physical therapy and supportive services are important aspects of MS management. Bladder symptoms should be evaluated by a urologist. Drugs are available that may alleviate incontinence or retention. Diet, adequate rest, and avoidance of temperature extremes, especially heat, are also important.

Polyneuropathy

Polyneuropathy affects the peripheral or autonomic nerves. Peripheral neuropathy may affect sensation, motor strength, or both in the hands and feet. Symptoms include numbness, tingling, and weakness. Symptoms of autonomic neuropathy include sweating, diarrhea or constipation, difficulty urinating, and impotence.

There are many causes of peripheral neuropathy, including genetic disorders, alcoholism or the abuse of other drugs, exposure to toxic substances, nutritional deficiency, metabolic disorders, inflammation, infection, chronic illness, and cancer. Peripheral neuropathy also may be a remote effect of cancer or a complication of chemotherapy. Guillain-Barré disease is a form of peripheral neuropathy. It is a viral infection characterized by progressive numbness and weakness. When it is severe, complete paralysis and loss of respiration may occur.

Diagnosis

Neuropathy is determined by a medical history and examination. Electromyography (EMG), a test of nerve and muscle function, is used to classify the neuropathy and pinpoint the part of a nerve affected. A nerve biopsy and special blood tests may be necessary.

Treatment

Treatment depends on cause. Some polyneuropathies, such as Guillain-Barré, are treated with plasmapheresis, intravenous gamma-globulin, or steroids. Recovery from Guillain-Barré may be complete, even in a severe case. Some genetic disorders are progressive. Physical therapy, adaptive equipment, and special shoes are sometimes necessary.

Tumor

Primary tumors of the nervous system originate there; secondary or metastatic tumors have spread from distant sites in the body. Primary brain or spinal cord tumors can be either benign or malignant; metastatic tumors are always malignant. Breast and lung cancers are especially likely to spread to the brain and spinal cord. Even a benign brain tumor may cause serious problems because of its size or inaccessibility to surgery.

Symptoms depend on the site affected. Headache, mental confusion, language impairment, visual change, weakness, or strokelike symptoms may indicate a brain tumor. Seizures may also be a presenting symptom. Spinal cord tumors cause back pain, difficulty walking, and bowel or bladder problems.

Diagnosis

Brain or spinal tumors are diagnosed by CT imaging or MRI. A pathologic diagnosis requires tissue confirmation, which may be done by a craniotomy, where the skull is opened, or by a stereotactic biopsy. A low-risk procedure when done by an expert, a stereotactic biopsy is done with the patient awake. A small hole is drilled into the skull and a probe is passed to the site to be biopsied, using the CT scan as a guide. Because the brain has no pain fibers, the procedure is not painful.

Treatment

Benign tumors are surgically removed unless their location precludes it. Malignant tumors may be treated with surgery, radiation, and chemotherapy, individually or in combination. Surgery is selectively used in cases of metastatic cancer.

Motor Neuron Disease

Motor neurons in the brain and spinal cord control movement. They are subject to a degenerative disease whose cause is unknown. Some cases are familial (inherited), and others may be the remote effects of a disease like cancer. Symptoms include a gradual wasting and weakness of muscles. All limbs are eventually affected. A bulbar form of the disease affects speech and swallowing. Mentation is always normal. There is no known treatment except in cases of remote effect where the cause is amenable to therapy. Progression is sometimes rapid, with death in 3 years due to respiratory failure. Others progress more slowly and are successfully managed with therapy, adaptive equipment, and portable ventilators for many years.

Myasthenia Gravis

A disease of the neuromuscular junction (the region between nerve and muscle) myasthenia gravis results in what is called fatigable muscle weakness. The term *fatigable* refers to weakness that occurs after repetitive use of a muscle, not to the generalized state of fatigue. Typically, the muscle weakness fluctuates during the day. Symptoms may be confined to the eye muscles, with complaints of droopy lids and double vision. Or the disease may involve facial, speech, and swallowing muscles, causing facial weakness and difficulty in chewing, swallowing and speaking. Involvement of limb muscles occurs in generalized myasthenia.

Peak age at onset in women is 20 to 30 and in men, ages 60 to 70. The disease rarely occurs in childhood.

Diagnosis

Myasthenia gravis is an autoimmune disease. It is due to a defect in neuromuscular transmission—antibodies form against receptors in the muscle membrane, decreasing the response to the neurotransmitter acetylcholine. Antibodies to the acetylcholine receptor are found in almost 90 percent of patients with generalized myasthenia, 70 percent of ocular myasthenia. The edrophonium (Tensilon) test and EMG are used for diagnosis. The edrophonium test, done in the doctor's office, consists of an injection of a drug that partially reverses the weakness. Patients with myasthenia are evaluated for thyroid disorders and for thymoma, a chest tumor. Pulmonary function tests are done to assess respiratory status.

Treatment

Treatment may include anticholinesterase drugs such as Mestinon, plasmapheresis, steroids, and immunosuppressive drugs. The thymus is removed (thymectomy) when a thymoma is present, unless medically contraindicated. In those cases without tumor, a thymectomy is usually recommended because there is good chance of remission following the procedure. Sometimes the disease spontaneously remits, but generally only for short periods. Myasthenia requires expert management and should be handled in centers where physicians have special expertise with the disease.

Degenerative Diseases

Dementia

Dementia, a gradual decline and loss of intellectual and social functioning, affects millions of Americans in their later years. One of the most common causes of dementia is Alzheimer's disease, which accounts for about 50 percent of all cases of dementia. The disease begins with a gradual loss of memory, increasing confusion and anxiety, and a growing irritability. The disease progresses to the point where the person is unable to work, socialize, or communicate. The disease is due to a degeneration of brain cells, but the exact process is unknown. To date, there is no effective treatment or cure. Other causes of dementia are stroke, brain tumor, head injuries, and some infectious diseases of the brain.

Amyotrophic Lateral Sclerosis (ALS)

Commonly called Lou Gehrig's disease, amyotrophic lateral sclerosis is a progressive degeneration of the nerve cells controlling voluntary motor functions. The symptoms include difficulty in walking; swallowing, speaking, or breathing problems; and a gradual wasting away of the muscles of the arms and legs. Death usually occurs within 2 to 10 years after diagnosis. The cause is unknown, and there is currently no effective treatment.

Huntington's Disease

Huntington's disease, or chorea, is a progressive hereditary disorder characterized by abnormal involuntary movements, personality changes, and mental deterioration. It is an autosomal dominant disease, which means the child of an affected parent has a 50 percent chance of inheriting the disease. The onset of symptoms is usually between 35 and 40 years of age, and death occurs within 10 to 15 years.

NEUROLOGICAL TESTS

Tests used to assess neurological disorders include imaging studies such as CT scans and MRI, plus tests that study the electrical impulses of the brain, tests of nerve and muscle function, and procedures to assess nerve responses to stimuli. Other procedures include an examination of cerebrospinal fluid and a biopsy of brain, nerve, and muscle tissue. The tests performed depend on the symptoms and the findings of an examination. Their purpose is to identify the area of the nervous system affected and to determine the cause of the problem.

Biopsy

A biopsy is a surgical procedure used to confirm a diagnosis. A piece of tissue is removed and studied under a microscope. In some cases, cultures are done to look for infectious organisms. A brain biopsy is done to determine the nature of a suspected tumor or to look for disease in brain tissue, such as infection or a degenerative process. A biopsy is often necessary because scans of different brain processes may look similar. A brain biopsy may be open (craniotomy) or stereotactic (done with a probe). The open surgical approach depends on the site and nature of the lesion. The risk is less for stereotactic biopsy, but the procedure may not work as well because of the small amount of tissue obtained. A nerve biopsy can provide information on nerve defects that may relate to inherited, inflammatory, or metabolic conditions. A muscle biopsy is part of the workup of patients with muscle weakness.

Electroencephalography

Electrical activity of the brain can be recorded on an electroencephalogram, which provides a picture of the functioning of the brain. Abnormal patterns can show up when the brain is not functioning properly. The test is especially helpful in seizure disorders and can be used to assess stuporous or comatose patients. It is also used to monitor the state of the brain under anesthesia during surgery, and in cases of injury or drug intoxication. A flat pattern, showing no brain activity, is accepted as brain death.

For the procedure, electrodes are placed on the patient's scalp and attached to a machine that produces a tracing. A sedative may be given before the test. There is no risk, and the test may be done on an outpatient basis.

Evoked Potentials

The stimulation of certain areas in the body can produce a response that can be traced by electrodes placed along nerve pathways. Electrodes are usually attached to the scalp, the responses are recorded on a graph, and the results are analyzed by a computer to show the pattern and strength of brain waves. Each peak or wave corresponds to a particular sensory relay, and alterations in the waves can show a problem at a specific site in the body.

Visual evoked potentials involve stimulation of the eye to detect problems in the optic nerve. The test can also be used to assess sight and blindness, particularly in the very young and the very old. Brain stem audio evoked potentials test hearing. A sound is made into an earphone, and the response is traced along the auditory nerve, inner ear, and parts of the brain that process sound. Somatosensory evoked potentials, used to monitor the spinal cord and brain stem, can help detect disorders or injuries, and may be used during surgery to ensure that these areas remain intact while being manipulated. The evoked potentials are also useful in patients with multiple sclerosis to detect delays in nerve transmission caused by loss of myelin.

Lumbar Puncture

The fluid that surrounds the spinal cord can show signs of infection, disease, bleeding, and pressure in the skull. A sample of fluid is obtained by placing a needle into the lumbar region of the spine through the membrane covering the spine (the dura). A local anesthetic is given before the procedure.

About 10 percent of patients have a headache following this procedure, and sometimes nausea and vomiting occur. Bed rest and a liberal intake of fluids are recommended to prevent post-lumbar puncture problems. In most patients, the symptoms resolve in a few days. In some, severe headache persists, called a post-lumbar puncture headache. This is due to persistent leaking at the puncture site, and can be treated with a blood patch, a minor procedure. Rarely, patients develop double vision, which is usually resolved in a few days or weeks.

Severe complications of lumbar puncture are uncommon. The procedure is safe and is usually performed in a doctor's office. There is no risk of injury to the spinal cord because the needle is inserted several segments below the termination of the cord. This test is contraindicated for patients with bleeding problems, large brain masses, and abscesses over the spine.

Imaging Studies

Several techniques are used for viewing the brain, spinal cord, and other areas of the body that relate to the nervous system. The test selected depends on the condition. Multiple tests are sometimes necessary.

Angiography

For this procedure, a catheter (tube) is placed into an artery and dye is injected through it. X-rays are then taken from different angles. This test can show a disruption or obstruction in the blood vessels, or the site of bleeding or an aneurysm. There is a small risk of neurological signs and symptoms of stroke, especially for patients with atherosclerotic disease, but these are usually transient. Other complications include an embolism, cutting or tearing of an artery, and an allergic reaction to the dye. The procedure is usually done in a hospital under the direction of a neuroradiologist.

Computerized Tomography (CT Scan)

This rapid and safe test provides images of the skull, cerebrospinal fluid, and brain. It can show structural defects, bleeding, fluid buildup, or tumors. Images of blood vessels can be enhanced and made clearer by intravenous injection of dye before the procedure. The technician takes pictures in small sequential slices, so that when they are reassembled by a computer, the image can show multiple planes. Risks are usually confined to dye reactions. A radiologist is present to treat such complications. The test can be done on an outpatient basis.

Magnetic Resonance Imaging (MRI)

For this test the patient is surrounded by a magnetic field through which pulses of radio-frequency radiation are projected. Coils are placed on or near the patient's body to serve as antennae in detecting changes caused by the radio-frequency waves. The information obtained from the coils is reconstructed by computer into an image. The test can show differences in tissue and bone structure and help identify masses. A contrasting dye is injected to show certain vascular details. (There is less risk of reaction to this dye than to the contrast used for a CT scan.) The test carries little risk and can be used during pregnancy without the dye. It cannot be used if a person has any metal in his or her body, such as metal clips or plates, or a pacemaker. It also may pose a risk with prosthetic devices, such as cardiac valves and orthopedic devices. The test can be done on an outpatient basis. The tubelike enclosure of the machine may cause a problem for those with claustrophobia. A mild sedative may help. "Open" machines are available, but picture quality may be compromised.

Myelography

In this procedure, dye is injected into the lumbar or cervical (neck) area of the spinal column to assess the spinal cord, blood vessels, ligaments, and discs. An X-ray and/or CT scan of the area is then done to obtain the image. The test is useful for showing compression of the spinal cord (as with a protruding disc), osteoarthritic bones, tumors, or abscess. Headache, nausea, and vomiting can occur but usually disappear within 24 hours. Seizures may occur but are rare. The procedure is thought to be relatively safe and is sometimes done on an outpatient basis or with an overnight hospital stay.

Nerve Conduction and Electromyography

This test is used to evaluate nerve and muscle function. For nerve conduction, a mild shocklike stimulus is applied to different nerves and an electrode record show fast the impulse travels along the nerve. Slowing, delay, and blockage of conduction can be identified. This test is useful in diagnosing carpal tunnel syndrome, Guillain-Barré, and other disorders that slow conduction.

For the electromyograph, fine needles are inserted into different muscles and are attached to leads. A pattern is generated on an oscilloscope that shows if there is a nerve problem, a muscle disorder, or both. Interpretation of the pattern is critical and requires an experienced physician, knowledgeable in muscle and nerve problems.

The test is mildly uncomfortable but not severely painful. It is done on an outpatient basis.

PART III

The Musculoskeletal System

Laura L. Tosi, M.D., F.A.A.O.S., and
Patience White, M.D., F.A.A.P., and
Judith J. Petry, M.D., F.A.C.S., and
Francesca Morosani Thompson,
M.D., F.A.A.O.S.

The bones that make up the skeleton, along with the muscles and connective tissues that bind them together, form the musculoskeletal system. This system provides a framework that allows the body to move. When the system is working properly, motion is full range and painless. Problems in the musculoskeletal system can restrict movement and affect daily living activities. Certain aspects of your lifestyle can affect the health of your musculoskeletal system. Seek medical advice if warning signs of problems occur, because some disorders can progress, becoming disabling and chronic if not treated.

STRUCTURE AND FUNCTION

Bones provide support for the body and anchor and protect the internal organs. The 206 bones come together at joints, which allow the skeleton to be flexible. The bones are connected at the joints by ligaments. Muscles, which are responsible for all movement, are attached to the bones by tendons. All the parts of the system work together to perform the thousands of acts that make up your capacity to move within your environment.

In addition to supporting the body and its organs, bones encase and protect certain organs. The skull protects the brain, and the rib cage shields the lungs and heart. Bones also serve as a storehouse for fat and minerals, the most important of which are calcium and phosphorus. Other minerals stored in the bones include potassium, sodium, sulfur, magnesium, and copper. These stored minerals are released into the bloodstream and are carried to all parts of the body as they are needed. Inside the bones is a cavity filled with soft, fatty, vascular tissue called marrow, which produces the oxygen-providing red blood cells, an important component of blood.

Each bone in the skeleton contains different proportions of two basic types of bone tissue called cortical bone and cancellous bone. Cortical bone is hard and dense, whereas cancellous bone has a honeycombed appearance similar to that of a sponge. Most bones in the female skeleton are the same shape as the bones in the male skeleton, but a little smaller. One exception is the pelvis. A woman's pelvis is usually broader than a man's and has a larger space in the middle. The shape allows for the head of a baby to pass from the uterus through the pelvis during childbirth.

The location where two bones meet is called a joint. The ends of the bones are covered with cartilage, which serves as a cushion between the bones. The joints are connected by fibrous tissue called ligaments and the joints are lined with a thin membrane called synovium. The synovial membrane produces fluid that provides nutrition for the cartilage and lubricates the joint, reducing friction and wear and tear (see box, page 107).

The joints are also cushioned by bursae. These sacs contain synovial fluid that helps prevent friction during activity. Bursae are located in areas of the body where ligaments, muscles, skin, or tendons rub against bone or against each other.

Ligaments attach bones together, and provide support for joints. The more ligaments located at a joint, the stronger it is. Joints are further strengthened by tendons that attach muscles to bone. The better the muscle tone, the stronger the joint.

Muscles are bundles of fibers or cells bound together by connective tissue. They are responsible for the movement of the body itself as well as the organs within the body. Muscles can translate messages from various parts of the body into mechanical energy to exert force. They also maintain posture and generate heat in the body to maintain normal temperature.

Muscle has the ability to contract or shorten when tensed, to extend or lengthen when relaxed, and to resume its original length after being contracted. Some muscles are voluntary (under conscious control) and others are involuntary (cannot be consciously controlled). There are three types of muscle:

- **Skeletal muscle** controls body movements on voluntary command.
- **Cardiac muscle** controls the involuntary beating of the heart.
- **Smooth muscle** controls the involuntary function of organs such as the stomach, urinary tract, and lungs.

Each skeletal muscle fiber has a nerve ending that controls its activity. To meet its energy needs, each muscle is served by an artery and one or more veins that circulate oxygen-rich blood to the muscle and remove byproducts. Each skeletal muscle is attached to bone or other connective tissue, such as cartilage or fibrous membranes, at a minimum of two points. Body movement occurs when muscles contract across joints, resulting in activity of the joint such as bending or stretching.

The skeleton—including bones, cartilage, joints, and ligaments—makes up about 20 percent of the body by weight. (See Fig. 3.1) Nearly 50 percent of the body's mass is muscle. These structures are made up of living, growing cells that renew damaged areas and change with age. Bone especially is subject to constant change as it is removed and replaced in a process called remodeling (see "Bone Remodeling").

During adolescence, a growth spurt changes the skeletal structure. The legs become longer, the hips and chest become wider, and the trunk lengthens. Skeletal growth stops around age 25. Around age 30, bone mass

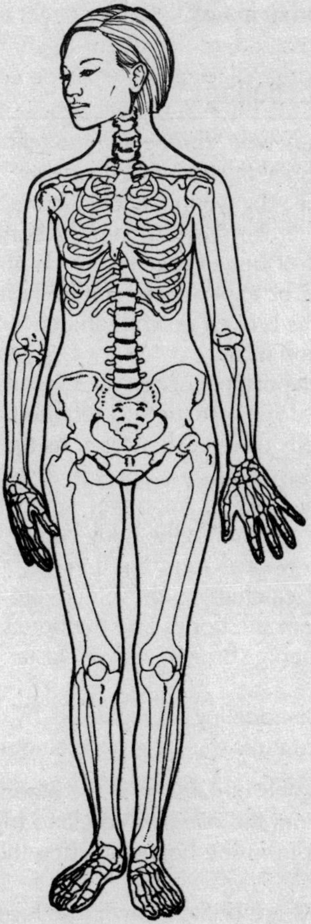

Figure 3.1 The Skeletal System
The skeletal system is made up of 206 bones. The hardest living tissue, bones provide a supportive framework, make movement possible, and are a source of calcium and red blood cells.

begins to decrease. The rate of bone loss is faster in females than in males.

Bone Remodeling

Bone is renewed through remodeling, a continual process of breaking down old bone and depositing new bone. In healthy young adults, bone mass stays the same; in other words the amount of bone deposited and the amount of bone broken down is about equal. As a person ages or experiences certain hormonal changes, more bone is broken down than deposited, resulting in a loss of bone mass.

Bone deposition occurs at sites of bone injury or where added bone strength is required. Bone is broken down by cells called osteoclasts. As the minerals in the bones are dissolved, calcium is released into the blood, serving a number of important functions in the body. Most of the calcium in the body comes from the bones. The body draws calcium stored in the bones as needed. If levels of calcium in the blood are low, it will be removed from the bones and the bones become weakened by being broken down faster than bone is replaced.

Bone remodeling is regulated by hormones in a cycle that controls the level of calcium in the blood:

1. When levels of calcium in the blood are low, a hormone from the parathyroid gland triggers release of calcium from the bones, causing the breakdown of bone.
2. As bones are broken down, the level of calcium in the blood increases. The thyroid gland then releases a hormone that halts the breakdown of bone and causes calcium to be removed from the blood and deposited in the bones.

3. As calcium is deposited in the bone, the level of calcium in the blood decreases. The parathyroid gland then signals an increase in the breakdown of bone so calcium can be added to the blood.

Bone remodeling is also affected by the amount of stress placed on bones. Stress can occur in the form of exercise, which strengthens bones. It is also exerted in the legs, ankles, and feet by the pull of gravity. Heavy use of bones results in increased bone deposits and heavier, stronger bones.

TYPES OF SYNOVIAL JOINTS

Synovial joints can be classified by how they function:

- Plane joints (hand and foot) allow slipping or gliding movements in all directions.
- Hinge joints (elbow, knee) move in only one direction.
- Pivot joints (forearm, head, and neck) allow rotation of one bone against another.
- Knuckle and saddle joints in the fingers and thumb, respectively, fit together to permit a wide range of movement.
- Ball and socket joints (shoulder, hip) are the most freely moving of joints.

KEEPING THE SYSTEM HEALTHY

The development of a strong skeleton begins early in life and can be affected by several factors, including exercise, diet (particularly calcium intake), and hormones.

The health of bones is affected by the amount of stress placed on them. The pull of muscles and gravity on bones makes then stronger and heavier. Good muscle tone also helps stabilize joints. Bones and muscles lose their bulk when they are not used, so it is important to exercise these vital parts of the musculoskeletal system to maintain its overall health. This is especially true for women, who have less bone density than men to begin with, and who are even more susceptible to bone loss in later life.

Bone mass, and the rate of bone formation and loss, can also be affected by diet. Calcium and vitamin D intake are needed throughout life in order to make bones strong enough to carry weight and resist breaking under stress. Both men and women gain fifty percent of their bone mass between the ages of 10 and 20. Adequate calcium intake of at least 1,200–1,500 mg of calcium each day in adolescence, combined with regular exercise, will promote a strong peak bone mass. Between the ages of 20 and 30 years, the bone mass increases only slightly. After age 30, bone loss begins to occur. Therefore, taking care to build strong bones in adolescence and young adulthood goes a long way to preventing osteoporosis later.

These dietary points are particularly important for women, because of their unique biological functions. Pregnancy and breast feeding require extra calcium. If a woman does not have adequate calcium in her blood, it is removed from the supply in her bones, thus weakening them. Smoking tobacco and drinking alcohol also promote bone loss. The hormone estrogen is responsible for regulating the woman's use of calcium from bone, promoting long bone growth, and helping to protect bone. However, the ovaries stop producing estrogen at menopause, hastening the loss of bone. This can lead to a condition called osteoporosis, or brittle bones that can break easily.

Osteoporosis in postmenopausal women can be slowed through exercise and increasing calcium intake to 1,500 mg/day. This can be accomplished by eating foods high in calcium, or by taking supplements. Hormone replacement therapy, or estrogen taken after menopause to replace that which is no longer being made by the ovaries, can also help prevent osteoporosis.

Osteoporosis can lead to hip fractures. A hip fracture is a break in the femur bone, just below the hip joint or in the upper thigh bone. Over 280,000 hip fractures occur in the United States each year, and most of these fractures occur in women. Women over the age of 65 have a 1 in 5 chance of suffering from hip fracture during their lifetime. Most hip fractures require extensive care, and many result in long-term disability and even death as a result of complications. In addition to taking steps to avoid osteoporosis, a woman should also try to make her home as safe as possible to prevent falls and accidents (See "Preventing Hip Fractures").

Exercise strengthens bones and decreases the rate of bone loss. To be most effective, the exercise should be weight bearing. Weight can be applied to the bones by the weight of the body, such as with walking, or by lifting or holding weights. Exercise also strengthens muscles and joints and helps make connective tissues more flexible.

Careful weight management is important to the health of the musculoskeletal system. Although heavier women have stronger bones, and thus are less at risk of osteoporosis, being overweight causes stress and strain on certain joints, especially the knees and hips. Women who have been overweight most of their lives are more likely to have a kind of arthritis called osteoarthritis, the gradual wearing away of cartilage and bone in the joints. Extra weight can also increase the pain involved with this condition.

The feet are the foundation upon which your whole body rests. They play an important role in the musculoskeletal system as well as in your overall health, comfort, and ease of activity. Proper foot care, including the selecting and fitting of shoes, can help prevent foot problems that plague many women.

Cancer can occur in bones just as it does in other parts of the body (see Part IV). It can begin in the bone or spread there from other areas. Because breast cancer often spreads to the bone, it's important to perform monthly breast self-examination and get regular checkups to detect breast cancer early, before it has spread.

As with many health problems, the first sign of a problem in the musculoskeletal system is usually pain. Any symptoms should be evaluated by a doctor, who may consult with a variety of health professionals, depending on the problem (see "Health Care Professionals").

Health Care Professionals

Health care professionals who treat disorders relating to the musculoskeletal system include the following physicians and therapists:

- *Orthopedic Surgeon*—a physician with advanced surgical training who specializes in the diagnosis and treatment of musculoskeletal disorders.
- *Physiatrist*—a physician who specializes in the evaluation and treatment of musculoskeletal and neurological diseases and conditions to effect rehabilitation of neuromuscular functioning (also called a specialist in Physical Medicine and Rehabilitation [PM&R]).

- *Rheumatologist*—a physician who specializes in internal medicine and has advanced training in rheumatology, which is devoted to diseases of the immune system and the musculoskeletal system, including the joints, muscles, and bones.
- *Physical Therapist*—a professional who helps patients return to normal musculoskeletal functioning following illness or injury.
- *Occupational Therapist*—a professional who helps patients achieve maximal independence in tasks of daily living after injury or illness.

Other specialists in related fields may be involved depending on the type of disorder:

- *Oncologist*—a physician who specializes in cancer, which can occur in bone primarily or spread there from other parts of the body.
- *Neurologist*—a physician who specializes in diseases relating to the nervous system, which can affect the musculoskeletal system.

OSTEOPOROSIS: PREVENTION AND TREATMENT

A gradual loss of bone mass, generally beginning about age 30, is a normal occurrence for both men and women. After growth is complete, women usually lose 30 to 50 percent of their bone density, while men lose 20 to 30 percent. If bone is no longer replaced as quickly as it is removed, a condition called osteoporosis develops, in which the bones become thin and brittle. This condition particularly afflicts postmenopausal women, who are often unaware that they have osteoporosis until a fracture occurs.

The exact medical cause of osteoporosis is not known, but a number of factors are known to heighten the risk, including a calcium-poor diet, physical inactivity, reduced levels of estrogen, heredity, excessive cortisone or thyroid hormone, being underweight, smoking, and excessive alcohol use. The disease can be prevented if your diet contains the necessary calcium and vitamin D during childhood, adolescence, and adulthood. The National Institutes of Health (NIH) recommend the following daily calcium intake:

11–24 years: 1,200–1,500 mg

Pregnant or nursing women 19 or older: 1,400 mg–2,000 mg

Before menopause: 1,000 mg

Menopausal, postmenopausal women not taking estrogen: 1,500 mg

Premenopausal, postmenopausal women taking estrogen: 1,000 mg

Vitamin D plays a major role in calcium absorption, so you should also increase your intake of this vitamin after menopause. Other recommendations to prevent osteoporosis:

- Exercise. You should engage in regular weight-bearing exercises, such as walking—one of the best methods of maintaining bone strength—jogging, hiking, tennis, bicycling, dancing, aquatic exercises, and weight training. The emphasis should be on an activity that combines movement with stress on the limbs. Start exercising slowly, especially if you have been inactive. Consult your doctor before beginning any exercise program.

- Maintain a healthy lifestyle. Eliminate smoking and excessive alcohol use; these cause bone loss and increase your risk of a fracture.
- Take medications to prevent further bone loss. Ask your physician about hormone replacement therapy, calcitonin, or other medications that will help to slow down the rate of calcium absorption in the body.
- Get medical help as soon as possible. If you think you are at risk of developing osteoporosis, consult your medical advisor. Treatment plans should be initiated as early as possible, because once bone is lost it is difficult to replace.

Preventing Hip Fractures

A broken hip, especially after menopause, is a serious injury. Although modern orthopedic surgical techniques and care can assist in healing of the bone, most hip fracture patients require extended periods of rehabilitation. They may need assistance from their family or home care, or may be transferred from hospitals to long-term-care facilities. Walking aids may be necessary for several months after the injury, and many patients will permanently require canes or walkers to move around the house or outdoors.

Who is at risk for hip fractures? For one, women over 65. Slender women with small bones may be more prone to such fractures than large, heavy-boned women, and a family history of fractures in later life is another important indication of vulnerability. Women who have a low dietary intake of calcium, smoke, or drink alcohol excessively are also in the higher risk category, as are those with arthritis, poor balance, coordination, and eyesight.

Obviously, prevention of hip fractures is far better, and far less costly, than treatment after the bone is broken. A diet high in calcium, regular exercise, and the correct medications can all help to prevent weak bones and the possibility of a hip fracture in the future. Remember, too, that most of these injuries occur as a result of a fall, usually in the home. There are steps that you can take to minimize your chances of such an accident:

- *Stairways.* Provide enough light to see each step clearly. Repair loose stairway rugs. Do not leave objects on the stairs. Install handrails on both sides of the stairway.
- *Bathrooms.* Install grab bars on the walls around the tub. Place a skid-resistant rug next to the bathtub for safe exit and entry. Use a nonskid rubber mat or textured adhesive strips on the tub and shower floor. Install a night light.
- *Bedrooms.* Place a lamp and flashlight near your bed. Keep the floor clear of clutter, and make sure the route between the bedroom and bathroom is clear of objects and illuminated by a night light.
- *Living areas.* Keep pathways clear of furniture, plants, lamps, and electrical cords and wires. Secure loose area rugs and runners with tape, tacks, or slip-resistant backing. Avoid standing on unsteady stools, chairs, or ladders to clean or to reach distant objects.

SIGNS AND SYMPTOMS

Problems in the musculoskeletal system usually appear first as pain. Pain can occur in the affected area or be felt elsewhere. This is called referred pain. Pain in smaller joints is usually more sharply localized, whereas pain in larger joints can be felt in a general area. Certain characteristics about pain aid in the diagnosis:

- Is the pain located in one spot, or does it occur all over the body?
- Does the pain involve one joint, or are several joints affected?
- Does the pain move from one joint to another, or has it steadily progressed to include several joints?
- Did the pain occur suddenly or develop over time?
- Has the pain become steadily worse, or does it come and go?
- How long has the pain lasted, and does it occur, worsen, or improve at certain times of the day?
- What factors make the pain better or worse?
- In what setting did the pain develop, and was it related to injury or excessive use of the body part affected?

In addition to assessing the nature of the pain and how it arose, related factors are considered in the diagnosis:

- Limitation in the normal range of motion of joints.
- Signs of inflammation, including swelling, tenderness in or around a joint, increased heat, or redness.
- Stiffness.
- Skin conditions or other symptoms occurring elsewhere in the body.

These signs and symptoms can help pinpoint the diagnosis. Their significance depends on the part of the body affected and the pattern of the symptoms. Treatment is based on the cause and can range from medication to surgery. Anti-inflammatory medications are often used in the treatment of musculoskeletal disorders.

Back Pain

The S-shaped curve of the spine makes it prone to problems. The backbone includes 24 individual vertebrae, as well as the sacrum and the coccyx at the end of the spine. (see Fig. 3.2) It is divided into three regions:

- Lumbar (lower back)
- Thoracic (chest)
- Cervical (neck)

The spinal cord runs through the middle of the spinal column. Nerves branch out from the spinal cord to the rest of the body. Thus, problems in the back can affect other parts of the body and cause pain.

Pain in the back is a frequent complaint. Fortunately, most back pain is the result of mild injuries or strains that are not serious and go away within a short time. In many cases, the cause of back pain is not

Figure 3.2 The Spine
The spine, or vertebral column, is made up of interlocking bones called *vertebrae*. The 26 bones of the spine include the 7 *cervical*, the 12 *thoracic*, and the 5 *lumbar* vertebrae. Five fused vertebrae form the single bone called the *sacrum*. The *coccyx* consists of two to four fused vertebrae that represent the tail of our prehuman ancestors.

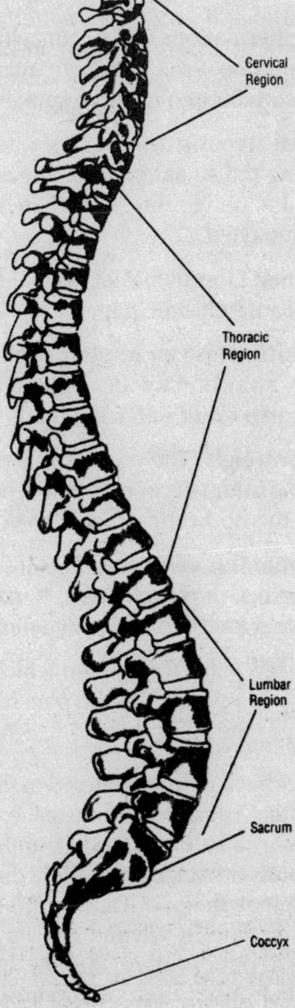
Cervical
Region
Thoracic
Region
Lumbar
Region
Sacrum
Coccyx

known. Conditions that may cause chronic back pain include:

- **Disc herniation:** This occurs when the fibrous cushion between vertebrae bulges out and causes pressure on one or more spinal nerves.
- **Spinal stenosis:** This occurs when the canal containing the spinal cord becomes narrowed, and thus the nerves traveling in the canal are squeezed and pinched.
- **Tumors:** Destruction of normal bone by tumors can cause chronic pain.
- **Arthritis:** This can result in joint surfaces being worn away and the development of bone spurs. Both can result in back pain.
- **Fibromyalgia:** The condition is characterized by aching and pain in muscles, tendons, and joints all over the body and especially along the spine.
- **Trauma:** This can cause fractures, injuries to the ligaments, or muscle tears. It may result in compression fractures of the vertebrae.
- **Referred pain:** This is pain which originates in other organs, such as the pancreas or kidney, but is felt in the back.

Lower back pain is centered in the small of the back and is often caused by unusual exertion or physical strain. It can also be caused by muscle spasms. Other causes of lower back pain include disc problems, arthritis, and spinal stenosis. Pain in the middle or thoracic part of the spine in women can be caused by muscle strain due to poor posture, fibromyalgia, or compression fractures that result from osteoporosis. Pain in the neck region is often related to disc problems and arthritis.

Back pain is cause for concern when pain or numbness travels down the legs, when bladder or bowel function is disrupted, or when the pain continues without improvement. The buttocks and legs may be affected. In some cases, pain may become more severe with coughing, sneezing, or bending.

Back pain is diagnosed by obtaining a history of symptoms, mapping the location and pattern of the pain, and physical examination. Additional studies may include X-rays, a computed tomography (CT) scan, magnetic resonance imaging (MRI), or bone scans.

Lower back pain may be treated with rest, moist heat, massage, and medication. Other treatments include weight reduction, exercise, and in some cases physical therapy and psychological counseling. Surgery is reserved for those patients in whom a treatable cause has been identified, such as disc herniation, or spinal stenosis.

Foot and Ankle Pain

Pain in the foot is often related to wearing improperly fitting shoes. Ill-fitting shoes can result in corns, calluses, and bunions, which are thickening and hardening of the skin over bony protrusions caused by friction. Wearing high heels can contribute to a condition called metatarsalgia, an inflammation of the metatarsal bones of the foot that causes pain in the ball of the foot. Another cause of foot pain is neuroma, in which swelling from a nerve causes pain between the toes.

Heel pain is caused by inflammation of the plantar fascia, a ligamentlike structure that begins at the heel and ends in the forefoot. In this condition, pain begins at the heel and extends along the arch of the foot. Problems relating to the Achilles tendon, which connects the calf muscle to the heel, can also cause pain.

This tendon can become inflamed or torn, usually as the result of an injury. Pain in the ankle is often due to sprains. The ligaments that support the ankle joint can become stretched or torn, usually as the result of a twisting injury. Severe pain, swelling, and bruising may occur.

The diagnosis of heel and foot problems depends on the location of the pain, whether it occurred in relation to an injury, and the nature of the pain. Usually the diagnosis is based on the results of an examination. An X-ray exam may be used to detect bone spurs or rule out fractures.

Hip Pain

Pain in the hip is a frequent complaint that can be hard to pinpoint. Pain from the hip can be felt in the groin area or the top of the thigh or the knee. Osteoporosis can lead to weakening of the bones and fractures, especially in elderly women. Pain along the outside of the hip can be caused by inflammation of the bursae located around the hip. If a disc in the spine presses on a nerve, it can cause sciatica, which can result in pain in the buttocks or pain radiating down the back of a leg. The location of the pain helps determine the diagnosis. In elderly women, hip fracture should be suspected, especially after a fall, even if they have only minor pain. If the fracture is unrecognized, it may become displaced (the bones may move out of place) and require more extensive surgery than might otherwise be required.

Joint Pain

Pain in a joint that is not swollen or inflamed is called arthralgia. Joint pain with inflammation and swelling is called arthritis. Certain disorders that result from infections, such as rheumatic fever, rubella, or Lyme disease, can cause joints to ache and become swollen. The autoimmune diseases, like lupus, can affect multiple joints. The pain can occur in a single joint, multiple joints, or move from one joint to another. Arthritis can be diagnosed by physical examination, blood tests, examination of the fluid from the joint, and imaging tests such as X-rays or MRI, and arthroscopy (direct viewing into the joint).

Leg and Knee Pain

Leg pain can be related to an injury or to muscle cramps. It can also be caused by problems in circulation, which are serious and should receive immediate medical attention. Shin splints are injuries that occur as a result of repeated pounding on hard surfaces, such as with jogging or tennis. The fibers that tie the muscle to the bone become inflamed and cause pain in the shin. They can be relieved through rest, applying cold, and elevating the injured area.

A muscle cramp is a spasm of the muscle that produces sudden and intense pain. It can occur as a result of muscle strain or as a result of overexertion, especially in warm weather when there is a risk of dehydration. Calf muscle cramps can also occur at night. Muscle cramps are not serious and usually can be relieved by gently stretching the affected limb. Massaging the muscle and applying heat, either in the form of a hot bath or heating pad, may also relieve the pain.

Pain in the knee is often the result of an injury, either new or old. Injuries commonly occur in athletic younger women. In older women, particularly those who are overweight, knee pain can be caused by osteoarthritis. Pain felt at the front of the knee, which can become worse when climbing stairs or exercising, can be caused by problems with the kneecap fitting into its groove and moving smoothly, a condition called chondromalacia patellae. It can also be caused by disorders in the cartilage and bone supporting the kneecap. Inflammation of the bursae, tendon, or synovial space in the joint between the thigh and calf bones can cause knee pain, as can a tear in the meniscus, the cartilage "washer" behind the knee cap that cushions the joint. (See Fig. 3.3) The diagnosis depends on how the pain arose and other symptoms present. Severe pain and fever could be a sign of an infection and should receive medical attention right away.

Shoulder and Elbow Pain

Pain felt in the shoulder is often referred from another area, such as the neck. A heart or lung problem can also cause shoulder pain. One of the most common musculoskeletal causes of shoulder pain is a condition called subacromial impingement, also known as rotator cuff tendinitis. The rotator cuff, the muscles and tendons that make up the shoulder joint, can become inflamed usually as the result of an injury or repeated motion. Injury or continued motion also can cause the rotator cuff to tear. The tendon that attaches the biceps muscle to the shoulder also can become inflamed as a result of repeated movement. If movement is constricted because of the pain, a "frozen" or severely limited shoulder may result. Although arthritis is not as common in the shoulder as it is in other areas, it can occur.

Pain along the outside of the elbow can be caused by small tears where the muscles are attached. This condition is called tennis elbow (or lateral epicondylitis), but it can occur for reasons other than playing tennis, mostly related to overuse or stress of muscles at the point of attachment to the bone. Grip strength is usually reduced and shaking hands with someone can be painful. The diagnosis is based on a physical examination, and treatment begins with rest and avoiding overuse. Exercises may be done to strengthen and stretch the forearm muscles, and wearing a forearm band or wrist splint may be helpful.

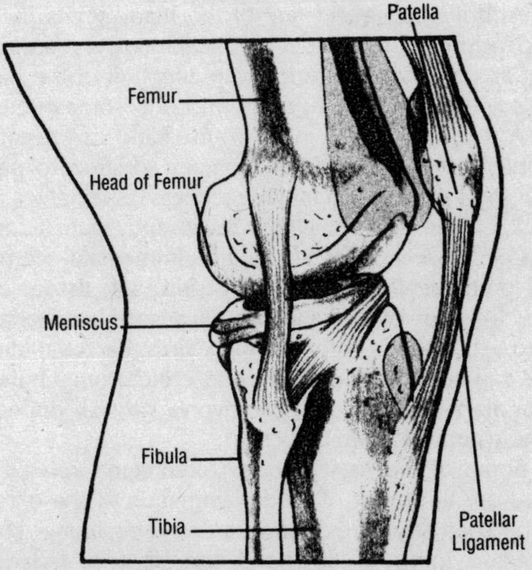

Figure 3.3 The Knee
The knee joint is one of the most complicated joints in the human body; it helps balance the entire weight of the body. It is surrounded by cartilage and ligaments that support it and allow movement. A crescent-shaped pad of cartilage, the *meniscus*, cushions the *femur*, or thigh bone, where it meets the *tibia*, the larger of the two bones in the calf and the stoutest bone in the body. (The *fibula*, the smaller of the two calf bones, forms part of the ankle joint.) The *patella*, or kneecap, is attached to the femur and tibia by the *patellar ligament*.

Hand and Wrist Pain

The hand is an intricate structure that is in constant use. The activities of everyday living subject the structures of the hand to repeated trauma. Pain in the hands can be caused by arthritis, infection, inflammation of the muscles and tendons, injuries, problems with circulation, or tumors. The complex and delicate anatomy of the hands complicates treatment of hand injuries.

Arthritis can affect any of the many joints in the hand, resulting in limited use. Inflammatory arthritis, such as rheumatoid arthritis, can affect all of the hand joints while osteoarthritis may affect only some of them.

A relatively minor injury to the hand can result in an infection that limits function. In addition to pain, other signs of infection include redness (especially a red streak on the arm), swelling, fever, and heat. If these signs occur, seek medical attention immediately to prevent permanent damage to the skin, soft tissue, and bone. Infection of the hand can be caused by bacteria or a virus, such as the herpes simplex virus. Bacterial infections can arise as a result of a bite, either from a human or an animal. Treatment may involve surgical drainage of the wound and antibiotics.

Some of the most frequent complaints related to hands are the result of the inflammation of these constantly used structures. Tendons and their lining, muscles, and joints of the hand can become inflamed through repeated use, causing pain and swelling. Tendinitis can occur with an unusual activity, such as painting, or as the result of an arthritic condition. Although it can occur anywhere in the hand, tendinitis most often occurs around the wrist. Muscles of the hand, particularly those in the fleshy part of the thumb, are subject to stress and can become swollen and painful. Severe swelling may rupture muscle fibers.

Pain in the wrist or hand can be caused by repeated use. Carpal tunnel syndrome, which causes pain, tingling, and weakness in the hand and wrist, results from compression of the median nerve. (see Fig. 3.4) Pain that occurs with movement of the thumb is often caused by a condition called DeQuervain's tenosynovitis, a condition in which the thumb tendons become inflamed.

Tendons and nerves of the hand are very close to the skin of the top of the hand, so a cut that appears to be minor can cause major damage. A cut on the finger

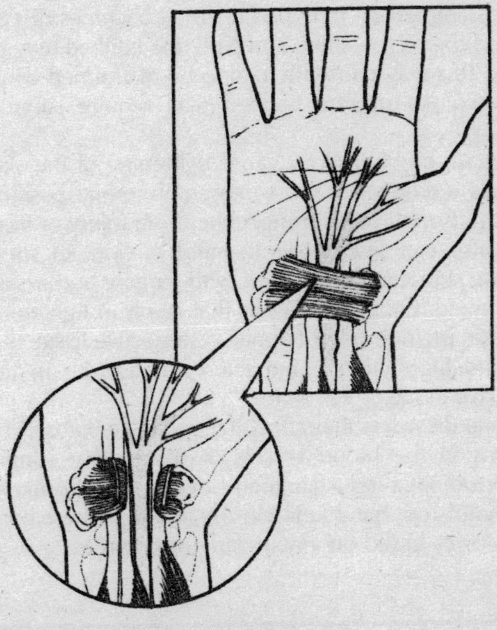

Figure 3.4 Carpal Tunnel Syndrome
Carpal tunnel syndrome is caused by compression of the *median nerve*, which runs through a sheath of muscle, the *retinaculum* ("carpal tunnel") at the wrist. The syndrome is common in pregnant women and in people who engage in repetitive hand and wrist movements.

or hand that results in the inability to bend or straighten the finger suggests that a tendon has been severed. Seek medical attention if any numbness, loss of motion, or severe pain on motion occurs after a laceration or cut. If a wound is dirty, it must be cleaned by a qualified health care professional. If a tendon or nerve has been injured, surgery may be required. Tendon injuries must be protected with a splint during healing. Physical therapy may be required to restore full function.

A fingertip may be crushed, such as when a car door is slammed on it; if the fingernail becomes discolored and there is swelling and pain, the nailbed may be injured. This may cause the nail to be malformed when it regrows. An injured nailbed may require surgical repair.

Certain problems can cause tightening of the skin that pulls the finger or wrist into an abnormal position and restricts motion. Scarring, either from injury or from burns, also can interfere with hand motion. In some cases the skin can be released with surgery and a skin graft applied. Other conditions that result in tightening of the skin include scleroderma, a connective tissue disease, and Dupuytren's contracture, a disorder in the connective tissue of the palm.

Some disorders that affect the hands are caused by problems in the blood vessels or nerves that supply them. A tumor called a ganglion can also arise from tendons and disrupt hand function. Treatment of these conditions varies based on any underlying disorder.

DISORDERS

Problems affecting the musculoskeletal system can either be limited to a specific area (usually due to an injury to that area) or can affect multiple areas. Such problems include infections, trauma, tumors, osteoporosis, certain medical disorders, and inflammatory conditions such as arthritis. Treatment is directed to the cause.

Achilles Tendon Injuries

The Achilles tendon links the leg muscles in the calf to the bone at the back of the heel. With exercise or strain, such as that which occurs with jogging or aerobic exercise, the tendon can become inflamed and even tear. Wearing high heels also may cause the tendon to become shortened, causing strain when the foot is flat. Symptoms include a dull ache or pain in the heel, especially with exercise. Swelling and tenderness may be noted as well. Since injury is usually the cause, the diagnosis is based on the patient's history and examination.

Treatment involves rest, applying ice to the ankle (when the injury is acute), and taking nonsteroidal anti-inflammatory drugs to provide relief. Occasionally a splint may be used. Heel lifts also may be used to raise the heel. Running or jumping is prohibited until the tendon has healed, then stretching and strengthening exercises can be done. If the tendon has ruptured or torn, it may have to be reattached with surgery.

Arthritis

Arthritis causes pain, swelling, and stiffness in joints. There are various types of arthritis based on the cause and the disease process involved. Some types of arthritis result from mechanical wear on the parts, whereas others occur for no known reason. Arthritis can also be caused by infections.

Osteoarthritis

Also known as degenerative arthritis, this condition is a chronic wearing away of the cartilage that protects the joint. With normal use, the cartilage in joints becomes worn, so many people develop osteoarthritis with age; osteoarthritis affects women more than men and usually occurs after age 40. Rarely, an injury, a birth defect, or overuse of a joint such as from being overweight may cause osteoarthritis at an earlier age.

Osteoarthritis may affect any joint in the body if there is a prior injury but is mostly found in the knees, big toes, and small joints at the ends of the fingers. Pain often occurs after using the joint and improves with rest. There is little or no morning stiffness and the joint may be swollen but is rarely hot or red. The disease is confined to the joints, so other symptoms usually are not present. The diagnosis is based on the history and physical examination. X-rays may help assess any damage to the joint. Treatment consists of applying heat to the joint, and weight reduction, particularly for arthritis in the knee and hip. (See Fig. 3.5) Exercises to keep joints mobile and to strengthen the muscles surrounding them may be helpful, and medications can be used for pain relief. Surgery to replace the hip or knee joint is occasionally required.

Rheumatoid Arthritis

This form of arthritis is a chronic inflammatory process that affects the lining of a joint, the synovium. It results in swelling and destruction of cartilage and bone over time. Women between the ages of 30 and 50 are most often affected. The cause of rheumatoid arthritis is not known. It could be related to a combination of inherited and environmental factors. It could also be an autoimmune disorder, by which the immune system mistakenly begins to attack specific tissues in the body.

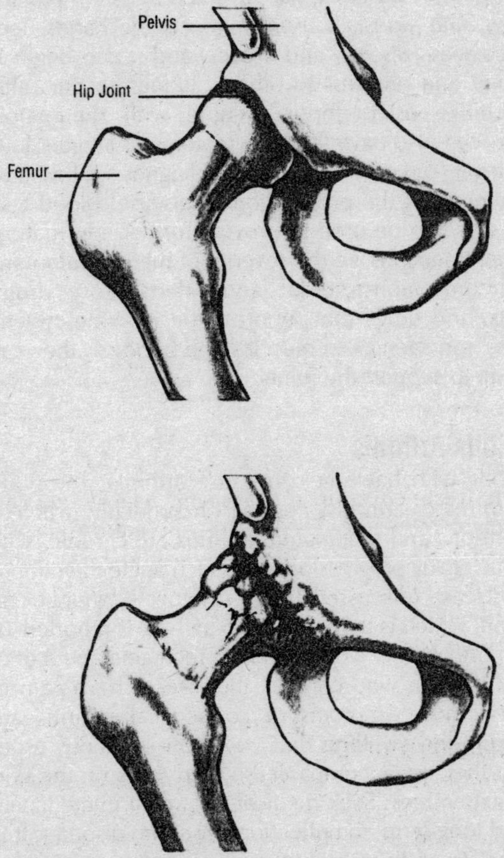

Figure 3.5 Arthritis of the Hip
Arthritis of the hip joint can cause a once healthy joint (top) to become painful as the cartilage is worn away and becomes scaly (bottom).

Like other forms of inflammatory arthritis, rheumatoid arthritis causes joints to become stiff, painful, swollen, and warm. It usually affects the hands, feet, wrists, knees, elbows, and ankles, and it can begin in one joint and progress to others. Stiffness occurs after rest. Unlike osteoarthritis, people with rheumatoid arthritis can also have flulike symptoms of fatigue, low-grade fever, and muscle aches. The diagnosis is based on the pattern and the progression of disease. Blood tests and X-rays can be used to provide further information. Treatment depends on the severity of the condition and can include nonsteroidal anti-inflammatory drugs, steroids, and drugs that suppress the immune system. Exercise can strengthen muscles and bones so they can continue to support the joints.

Infectious Arthritis

Infections with bacteria can cause arthritis. These are acute forms of arthritis, coming on suddenly, whereas osteoarthritis and rheumatoid arthritis are chronic, with slow but steady progression. One such acute infection is Lyme disease (discussed later). Another is gonococcal infection, which is transmitted sexually. It is reported 10 times more often in women than in men, and about one-third of women who contract the disease have pain in several joints. Symptoms of gonococcal arthritis are joint pain and swelling that come on suddenly, especially if they are accompanied by red sores on the skin of the extremities. Seek medical treatment immediately to avoid long-term complications from the disorder. It is treated with antibiotics. Both sexual partners must also be treated and should abstain from sex until treatment is completed.

Bursitis

A bursa is a saclike structure near areas of the joints that are subject to heavy movement. Bursae cushion the tendons moving near joints and help reduce the amount of friction. Bursitis occurs when the bursae become inflamed because of strain or injury. Repeated physical activity, such as swinging motions involved in tennis, golf, or baseball, can lead to bursitis. Most commonly, it can affect the shoulder, knee, elbow, or hip. Pain and swelling can occur at the affected area or near a joint as fluid accumulates in the bursa. The diagnosis is based on a physical examination and assessment of recent activities. During the examination the doctor can locate the area of tenderness and swelling and check the range of motion of the joint. Diagnostic X-rays may be taken to detect any other causes or to show old injuries.

Drugs such as a nonsteroidal anti-inflammatory will ease the pain, and often bursitis disappears on its own within a few weeks. If it persists, however, some of the fluid may be removed from the bursa with a syringe to relieve the pressure. Corticosteroids may be injected directly into the bursa in the area of the affected joint or, rarely, it may need to be removed by surgery.

Compression Fractures

These fractures can occur with minimal injury, often because bones are weakened by osteoporosis. The most common cause of back pain in the thoracic region is compression fracture due to osteoporosis. About one in every four women has a vertebral fracture by the time she reaches age 60. (See Fig. 3.6)

A woman may lose height as a result of compression fractures of the spine. She may feel pain in the middle of the back, but often there are no symptoms. The

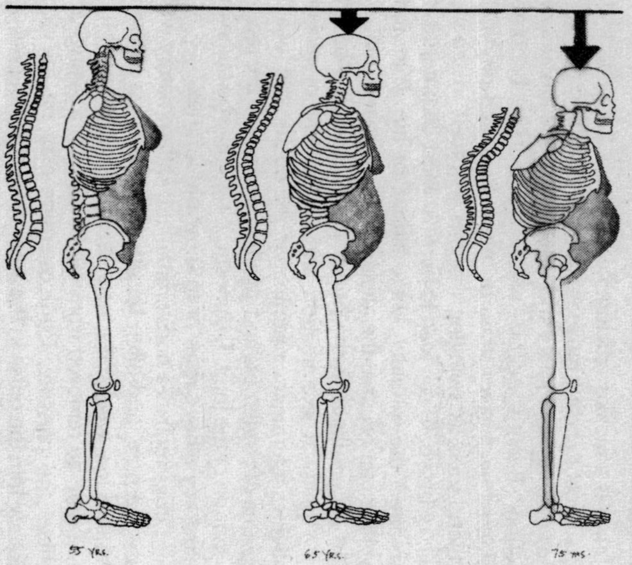

Figure 3.6 Osteoporosis
Osteoporosis causes bone mass to be lost, which can result in compression fractures in the spine. As normal vertebrae (left) begin to lose bone mass and weaken under the body's weight (middle), the spinal column collapses and shortens (right), causing the characteristic "dowager's hump" seen in individuals with this condition.

condition is diagnosed by X-rays. There is no cure for osteoporosis, but its progress can be slowed through diet high in calcium, exercise that strengthens the bones and helps prevents bone loss, and hormone replacement therapy.

Disc Problems

Discs are pieces of cartilage between the spinal vertebrae that separate and cushion the vertebrae as you move. A disc can be ruptured when injury, compression fractures, or wear and tear cause the gel-like center to squeeze against the spinal cord or one of the nerves. When this occurs, the disc is said to be herniated, prolapsed, or "slipped." This is most likely to happen in discs in the lower back and neck, although it can occur in any of the vertebrae in the spine.

A prolapsed disc in the lower back may arise acutely from an injury such as lifting. A woman often reports she felt a sudden "snap" in her low back while performing a task. In other cases, the symptoms may come on gradually. Pain may be felt in the lower back only or in the buttock and travel down the thigh and leg. This type of pain is called sciatica because it is felt along the course of the sciatic nerve. A prolapsed disc in the neck may cause sudden, extreme pain in the neck that is made worse by moving the neck, coughing or straining.

As a woman ages, her discs gradually dry out and lose elasticity. The bones of the neck may respond to this by forming spurs known as osteophytes. This combination is called cervical spondylosis. It can cause the spinal cord, as well as spinal nerves, to be compressed. This can result in pain with movement of the head, which can radiate to the shoulders, upper extremities, and chest area. Reflexes and sensations may also be affected.

Spinal stenosis occurs in the lumbar spine when the channel that holds the spinal cord becomes narrowed by thickened ligaments, breakdown of the vertebrae, and protruding discs. This can cause pressure on multiple nerves and result in pain in the legs and back after prolonged standing or walking. The pain can be on one or both sides and can go deep into the thigh. Other symptoms, such as weakness, loss of feeling in the legs, or urinary problems, also may occur.

A prolapsed or herniated disc is diagnosed based on symptoms and clinical findings on examination. The nature of the symptoms depends on the disc and nerves affected. If a prolapsed disc is suspected, a CT scan or MRI of the neck or spine can locate the area where the disc is out of place. Treatment depends on the disc affected and whether there are signs of nerve damage. A prolapsed disc in the neck is treated by immobilizing it with traction, or resting on a collar and giving medication for pain and muscle spasms. A prolapsed disc in the lumbar region is treated with bed rest and pain medication. Surgery may be required if the condition does not improve or there are signs of neurologic impairment.

Dupuytren's Contracture

This disease of the palm causes the fingers, especially the ring and small finger, to be gradually pulled into the palm. The disease causes a shortening, thickening, and hardening of the connective tissue just under the skin of the palm. There is a tender lump in the palm, which may progress to becoming a cord that extends to the fingers. The cause of the disease is unknown, but it runs in families and seems to be associated with epilepsy, diabetes, injuries, and alcoholism.

If a finger is left in the bent position, the joint stiffens. Surgery is indicated when one or more fingers cannot be straightened completely. It involves removal of the diseased tissue to release the fingers. Although surgery has a high success rate, the disease may progress to other fingers.

Fibromyalgia

This condition affects more women, especially those over middle age, than men. The cause of the disorder is unknown, but those women who don't get enough deep or rapid eye movement (REM) sleep seem to be at higher risk.

Aching and pain occur in the muscles, tendons, and joints all over the body. The condition often affects the back and can cause muscle tenderness. The pain may take the form of a tingling sensation. The joints don't swell but may feel stiff. Multiple tender spots are located along the spine and the extremities. The condition is associated with extreme fatigue and sleep disturbance, which may be severe.

The diagnosis is based on the history, excluding other causes of these symptoms, and treatment is with sleep-promoting drugs, nonsteroidal anti-inflammatory drugs, and lifestyle changes involving a reduction of stress, exercises, and relaxation techniques.

Foot Problems

Many foot problems in women are caused by ill-fitting shoes. The most common problems are bunions, corns, and calluses. In some women, arthritis can occur in the joint of the big toe, causing extra bone to pile up at the joint and produce pain. Most of these problems can be prevented or helped by proper footwear.

Bunions

A bony protrusion on the outside of the joint at the base of the big toe occurs when pressure is concentrated on the big toe, changing the normal profile of the foot. Over time, the big toe may turn sideways so you are walking on the bony inner side of the toe instead of the bottom, where the padding is. (See Fig. 3.7) The bunion is often subjected to constant rubbing, which results in a thickening of the skin (callus) and pain. The cause of bunions is usually wearing shoes that are too narrow. The best therapy is wearing shoes that have ample room for toes and that do not put pressure on them. (Fig. 3.8) When shoe changes do not relieve the bunion pain, surgery may be considered.

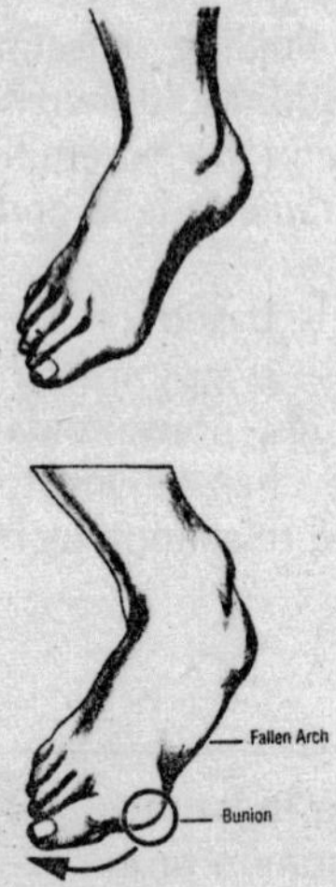

Figure 3.7 Bunions
Bunions are bony protrusions that form on the joint at the base of the big toe. A normal-appearing foot (top) can become bent (bottom), so that weight is placed on the inner part of the foot, causing the arch to collapse.

Corns and Calluses

Constant pressure or repeated friction on the skin produces a thickening and hardening of the skin. This often occurs on and between the toes, causing discomfort. Some women get hard calluses, called corns, on the top of their toes or soft calluses between their toes. Corns are often associated with hammer toes and claw toes, when the toe becomes permanently bent from being in that position. Corns and calluses on the feet are usually caused by poorly fitting shoes and high heels, and can be relieved by wearing soft shoes of the proper shape. The thickened skin of corns can be gradually removed with a towel or mild abrasive (such as a pumice stone or file) after it has been softened by a shower or bath. If the problem persists, the tissue may need to be removed surgically.

Neuroma

This condition involves a painful swelling of a nerve located between two toes, usually between the second and third or third and fourth toes. It arises from excessive pressure inside the foot. Symptoms include intermittent burning pain between the toes, particularly

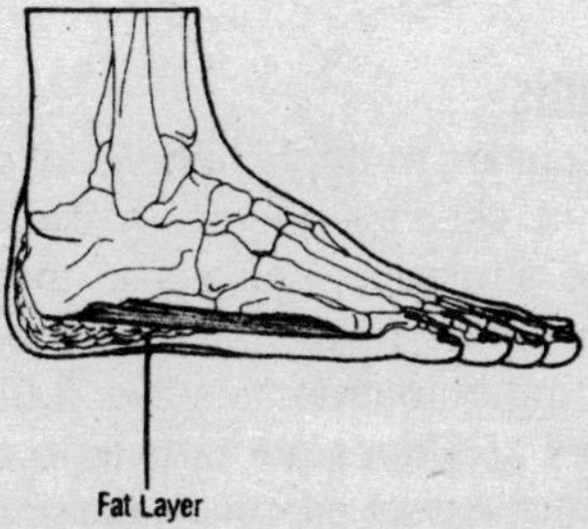

Figure 3.8 Foot Padding
The foot is padded at the heel with a layer of fat that helps cushion the impact of movement.

while bearing weight. Pain can become worse with running or walking, and may be eased by sitting down, removing the shoe, and rubbing the foot. The diagnosis is based on a physical examination. Treatment may involve pads under the ball of the foot to cushion it, nonsteroidal anti-inflammatory drugs, and steroid injections. Relief is usually obtained by widening the shoe, lowering the heel, and softening the insole. Rarely, surgery may be required to remove the growth if the pain is disabling.

Metatarsalgia

This is aching pain felt directly under the bones of the forefoot, especially when weight is placed on the foot. It is usually related to too much pressure being placed on the metatarsal part of the foot, often the result of wearing thin soled or very high-heeled shoes. The diagnosis is based on an examination. Therapy is oriented toward unloading the pressure on the metatarsals by wearing a cushioning pad or a custom-molded shoe with a pad. Shoes with ample room for the toes allow weight to be evenly distributed over all the metatarsals so they can share the weight. This condition can also be caused by arthritis in the metatarsal area.

Plantar Fasciitis

The plantar fascia are multiple bundles of connective tissue arranged in sheets underneath the foot. Chronic strain on these structures can cause them to become inflamed. Bone spurs of the heel may occur as a by-product of the inflammation. (See Fig. 3.9) Pain is localized to the heel and does not radiate to the rest of the foot. It is usually most severe on awakening or at the end of a long day of standing or walking. The heel is tender to the touch, especially if the first toe is extended.

The diagnosis is usually established by an examination. An X-ray may reveal a bone spur. Treatment is usually nonoperative and includes nonsteroidal anti-inflammatory drugs, heel stretching, rest, decreased weight bearing, and cups to cushion the heel. Steroids may be used, but multiple injections may cause atrophy of the heel pad. Surgery to remove a bone spur or release the plantar fascia may be required.

Ganglion

A benign (noncancerous) tumor that occurs on a tendon or at a joint, a ganglion is a thin fibrous capsule enclosing clear fluid. It ranges in size from a pea to a golfball and often appears in the hands and wrist, although it can occur in other places as well. It may occur as a

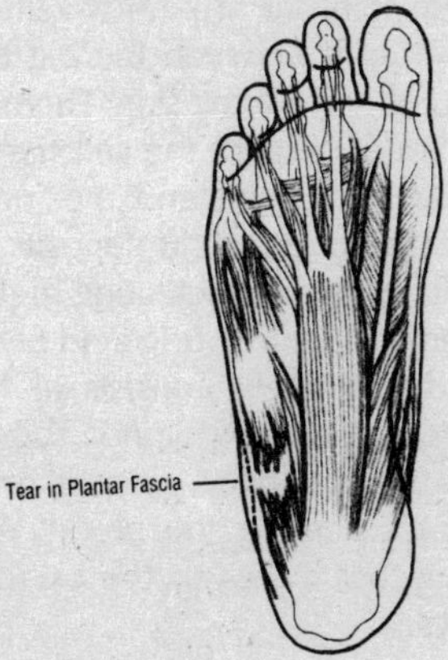

Figure 3.9 Foot Pain
A tear in the *plantar fascia*, the wide ligament that stretches from the heel to the front of the foot, can cause inflammation, pain, and swelling.

result of an injury or repetitive strenuous wrist activity, but often there is no apparent cause. Discomfort may be caused by pressure on adjacent structures. A ganglion may go away on its own. A large painful ganglion can be treated by removing fluid from its center with a needle, or removing it with surgery. It may recur, however.

Gout

This condition occurs when uric acid, one of the body's waste products that is normally passed out of the body through the urine, builds up in the blood and is deposited in the joints. It is inherited, and it can be worsened by high-protein diet and overconsumption of alcohol. It can also be caused by some medications. Uric acid crystals cause inflammation in the joints and can accumulate in the kidneys and urine, causing kidney stones. Symptoms include sudden onset of pain, swelling of a single joint (usually the joint between the big toe and the foot), and redness of the overlying skin. There can be a fever. If the disease is not treated, the soft tissue may become inflamed around the joint and the joint may become deformed because of uric acid deposits.

The condition is diagnosed by detecting high levels of uric acid in the blood and finding uric acid crystals in a sample of joint fluid. Treatment consists of NSAIDs (not aspirin) or a drug called colchicine. Those who experience recurrent attacks can be given a drug that lowers the levels of uric acid in the blood. Another option is to take a drug that increases the excretion of uric acid by the kidneys.

Infections

Infections of the bone—called osteomyelitis—have become increasingly rare because of the widespread availability of antibiotics. Before antibiotics were available, chronic infection of the bone (often as a result of trauma) or of the joints (as a result of tuberculosis) were crippling and sometimes fatal. Today chronic infection of bone usually occurs after a compound fracture, when a broken bone punctures the skin. When this occurs, the ends of the bone can die and lose their blood supply. Bacteria can live here easily and multiply quickly. Because of the poor blood supply to the bone ends, antibiotics cannot reach the bone easily. For this reason, open fractures are treated with thorough cleansing in the operating room to prevent infection. Similarly, an orthopedic operation can interfere with the blood supply of bones. Antibiotics are used to prevent infection after surgery.

Other types of infection can also cause problems in the musculoskeletal system. Certain types of bacterial infection cause arthritis. These include gonococcal infections, which are sexually transmitted, and Lyme disease, which is carried by ticks (see "Arthritis" and "Lyme disease").

Gangrene

This infection of the muscle usually occurs from an open wound. It spreads rapidly and produces toxic effects throughout the body that, if untreated, can cause severe illness. Symptoms usually occur 2-4 days after the wound, and the first symptom is sudden and severe pain at the site. The diagnosis is based on clinical findings and identification of the infecting organism. Treatment involves giving antibiotics and removing the infected tissue with surgery.

Lyme Disease

This disease is named after the location in Lyme, Connecticut, where it was first discovered in 1976. Since then it has spread rapidly and is now most prevalent in New England, New York, New Jersey, and areas of the Mid-Atlantic and the Mid-West. Lyme disease is caused by a spirochete (a type of bacteria) infection of the blood that spreads to the connective tissues and causes symptoms of arthritis. The bacterium is carried by a deer tick, which lives on a variety of animals, including deer, mice, and dogs and cats that are outside. The tick is smaller than a regular tick and thus can be hard to detect.

Lyme disease can have three phases:

- Early localized infection: A red mark can form at the site of the bite. The rash can then spread to cover the entire back or leg. The rash is present in about one quarter of those affected and often disappears within a few days. General flu-like symptoms of fatigue and nausea often are present.
- Early disseminated infection: A rash may occur. The heart muscle may become inflamed and cause an irregular heartbeat. Nerves, especially the facial nerve, may be affected, resulting in paralysis or a condition called Bell's palsy.
- Persistent infection: Sixteen weeks or more after the initial infection, arthritis can occur. Areas most affected include knees, shoulders, elbows, ankles, and wrists, in that order. The joint of the jaw also may be affected. Up to 10 percent of patients can develop chronic arthritis in one or both knees, even after treatment.

However, someone with Lyme disease may proceed from the early stage to the persistent phase of the illness and be completely asymptomatic. Similarly, individuals with Lyme disease may first develop symptoms at the early localized, early disseminated, or persistent phase.

Most patients develop antibodies to the infection within 6 weeks after they are exposed to it. Although antibodies are usually produced by the body to prevent it from further infection, these antibodies do not seem to offer future protection against this disease.

The best way to protect against Lyme disease is to prevent tick bites. Use insect repellents containing DEET and wear long pants, preferably white ones that will show the ticks, when hiking through grass. The ticks are often brushed off deer and stay on tall grass. Check yourself and your children regularly for ticks and remove them promptly, making sure to remove both the head and the body. Use tweezers.

If symptoms develop, consult a doctor as soon as possible. Tests can be performed to detect the antibody to the infection. Unfortunately, current laboratory tests are not perfect in diagnosing the disease. Also, since it takes 6 weeks for antibodies to develop, the test will not be positive until that time.

Lyme disease is treated with antibiotics. In early localized infection with a rash, a 2–3 week course of treatment is usual and will prevent progression of the disease. In persistent infection, longer courses of oral or intravenous antibiotics may be required.

Medial Meniscus Tear

The medial and lateral menisci of the knee are half-moon shaped wedges of cartilage that act as a buffer or bumper in the joint between the thigh and the shin bones to soften the force of weight on that joint. The meniscus can tear from trauma or a sudden twisting injury of the knee. When this occurs, there is severe pain over the inside of the knee and swelling that does not go away quickly. The condition is diagnosed by physical examination and MRI. Surgery may be required to repair or remove the meniscus. Arthroscopic surgery has had a major impact in improving the management of this problem.

Osteoporosis

Osteoporosis is a condition that results in bone loss with aging. (See Fig. 3.10) As a woman's bones become weakened, she is susceptible to fractures, which can

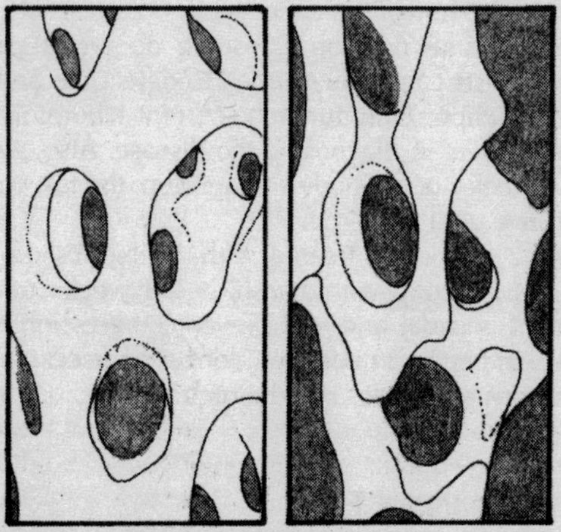

Figure 3.10 Osteoporosis
Osteoporosis is a condition in which normal bone (left) begins to lose the cells that produce new bone. This results in decreased bone mass, giving the bone a spongy appearance (right). Osteoporosis is more common in women than in men because of the natural decline in the hormone estrogen, which plays a role in bone cell production, that occurs with menopause.

occur with only minor injury. Osteoporosis can lead to compression fractures of the vertebrae and back pain, particularly in the thoracic region of the back. It can also increase the risk of hip fractures, which should be suspected if hip pain is present, even if a woman cannot recall an injury. If the hip fracture is not displaced, that is, if the bones are still in place and have not moved—the fracture is relatively easy to treat. If not treated, however, a hip fracture can become displaced and require major surgery to repair. Treatment can involve placing a pin in the hip to hold it in place or replacing part or all of the hip joint.

Osteoporosis can be slowed through exercise, a diet high in calcium, and hormone replacement therapy. Back pain related to osteoporosis can be improved through the use of nonsteroidal anti-inflammatory drugs and exercises that strengthen the back muscles. With any pain, particularly in the wrist, collarbone, or hip, a fracture should be suspected, especially in older women.

Paget's Disease

In this disease, new bone is produced faster than old bone is broken down. The new bone is more spongy than compact, which leads to weakening of the bones. As new bone continues to be produced and old bone is not broken down, the bones may become thickened and the bone marrow cavity filled. The cause of this disorder is unknown, but it may be linked to a viral infection. It may affect many parts of the skeleton but is usually localized to the spine, pelvis, femur, and skull, which can become deformed and painful. The condition can be diagnosed with blood tests and X-rays. Treatment focuses on medications that strengthen the bones and relieve pain.

Polymyalgia Rheumatica

This disease of unknown origin affects people over 50, especially women. It causes pain in the hip and the shoulder regions and may be associated with a general sensation of not feeling well, weight loss, and fever. Symptoms of aching and stiffness may come on suddenly.

This condition may be related to another called giant-cell arteritis, or temporal arteritis. The temporal artery, which passes just in front of the ear and across the temple, becomes inflamed and interferes with the blood supply to the optic nerve. Blindness can result if the condition is not treated promptly. The first sign of this arthritis is a headache that recurs and is usually more severe on one side. Scalp tenderness also may be noted, and the artery may be enlarged.

Polymyalgia rheumatica is diagnosed by history, physical examination, and blood tests. If giant-cell arteritis is suspected, a biopsy of the artery may be performed. Complications can be avoided by early diagnosis and treatment with nonsteroidal anti-inflammatory drugs (NSAIDs) and/or corticosteroids.

Polymyositis

These disorders of unknown cause affect the muscles and connective tissue, and some types are much more common in women. The disorder may have an autoimmune or genetic cause or be related to a viral infection. Symptoms can begin slowly and include weakness in the hip or shoulder muscles. In some cases, symptoms can come on suddenly and include fever or skin rash, rapidly progressing muscle weakness, and pain and tenderness. This disorder is diagnosed based on the physical findings, laboratory tests to detect muscle enzymes in the blood, electromyography to measure electrical responses of muscle contraction, and muscle biopsy to look for changes in the cells. The goals of treatment are to suppress the inflammatory response and reduce the loss of muscle and its strength. Results are best when treatment is given in the early stages. Treatment consists of corticosteroids or drugs that suppress the immune response. Physical therapy can teach patients exercises that reduce weakness and shrinking of muscles.

Raynaud's Disease

A disorder of the blood vessels, Raynaud's disease affects 3-4 times as many women as men. The symptoms are related to exposure to the cold and emotional stress, which cause pain, numbness, and a bluish or white color to the fingers and toes. Once the area is rewarmed, it is very pink for a time until normal color and sensation return. The spasmodic narrowing of the blood vessels that occurs with this disorder decreases blood flow and can lead to the development of ulcers or infection of the skin. Raynaud's disease can occur along with other disorders, such as scleroderma, lupus erythematosus, and arthritis.

Drugs that increase blood flow to the fingers and prevent the abnormal narrowing brought on by cold and emotional stress can be very effective in limiting attacks. The condition also can be treated with surgery of the nerves, but it is not always effective and complications are common. When Raynaud's disease is associated with other diseases, both problems must be treated.

Reflex Sympathetic Dystrophy

This is a poorly understood, disabling condition that can occur after what appears to be minor injury or surgery. It can occur in any extremity, and may be associated with overactivity of nerves that control the opening and closing of blood vessels and regulation of skin temperature. Symptoms include burning pain, swelling of the extremity, sweating, bluish discoloration, and stiffness. Treatment consists of nerve blocks or biofeedback to regulate the nervous system, physical therapy, and medication.

Scleroderma

A connective tissue disease that affects many organ systems, scleroderma involves the progressive replacement of normal tissues by dense, thick, scar-like tissue. The cause is unknown. It occurs most often in women between the ages of 30 and 40. In early stages, scleroderma can appear in the hands as tight skin limiting mobility. In later stages, the skin becomes increasingly thick and tight, hair and the ability to sweat are lost, and the skin may have the consistency of wood. Years after this stage has been reached, the skin may soften again. The treatment for scleroderma of the skin includes daily exercise of all joints, keeping the skin moisturized, and some specialized medications. Without proper treatment, the disease can affect interior organs, often fatally.

Spinal Curvature

The normal spine curves gently backward (kyphosis) in the upper back and gently inward in the low back (lordosis). However, there are several conditions that cause exaggeration of the normal curvature. Some are present at birth and some result from disease, poor posture, and the effects of aging. If very severe, abnormal spine curvature can interfere with movement and with body functions such as breathing. Mild cases are common, however, and may not require treatment.

Lordosis

When exaggerated, this condition is also called "swayback." It can be caused by disease, but more commonly results from abnormal weight distribution, such as with pregnancy or obesity.

Kyphosis

Also known as "roundback," kyphosis is an exaggerated rounding of the normal part of the spine. It can worsen during adolescence or it can result from compression of vertebrae that occurs with aging, particularly with women who have osteoporosis. It can also occur as the result of disease.

Scoliosis

An abnormal curving of the spine to the side, most often in the thoracic or thorocolumbar region. It commonly appears during adolescence, especially in girls. Although most progression of the curve occurs prior to the end of growth, severe curves can continue to progress during adulthood. (See Fig. 3.11) In severe cases, a body brace or surgery is needed before growth ends to prevent deformity or breathing problems.

Systemic Lupus Erythematosus

An autoimmune disorder in which the body's immune system attacks healthy cells, lupus can cause inflammation throughout the body. It can affect the skin, kidneys, lungs, heart, and nervous system, as well as the musculoskeletal system. The condition is much more common in women than in men, and usually occurs between the ages of 15 and 40, although it can occur at any time. Those who have a family history of the disorder are more at risk, and it may be linked to hormonal or environmental factors.

Systemic lupus erythematosus causes aching and swelling in the joints, often accompanied by fever, weight loss, and morning stiffness. Other symptoms include a butterfly-shaped rash on the face, chest pain, hair loss, swelling of the legs, high blood pressure, and depression.

People who have lupus have certain antibodies circulating in their blood. The diagnosis is based on the history, the symptoms, and the presence of these antibodies. The condition can get better or worse over a period of years. Therapy is directed toward suppressing inflammation and relieving symptoms. Treatment varies

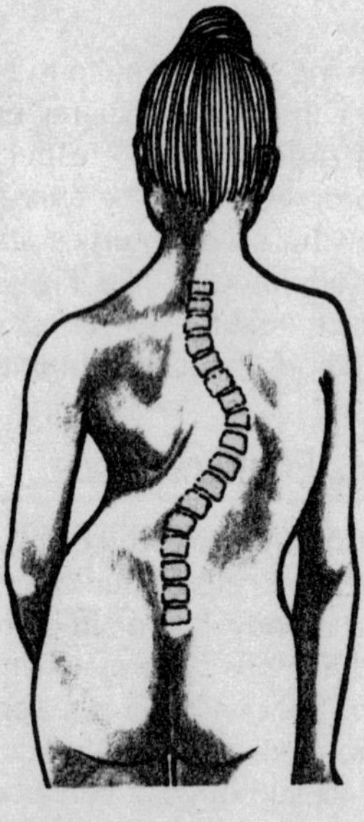

Figure 3.11 Scoliosis
Scoliosis, or curvature of the spine, has a number of possible causes, including abnormalities of the vertebrae, weakness of the muscles that support the spinal column, and inherited birth defects.

depending on the organ system involved and may include NSAIDs, corticosteroids, and drugs that suppress the immune system.

Tendinitis

Tendinitis is an inflammation of the tendons, the fibrous cords that attach the muscles to bones, usually caused by injury or overuse. It causes painful tenderness over the affected area, and the tendon is usually slow to heal because the muscle is in constant use. The area can become stiff because of the natural tendency to favor a painful area by not exercising it. Tendinitis often occurs in the shoulder in the form of rotator cuff tendinitis. It can also occur in the elbow (tennis elbow), and in the wrist.

Physical examination confirms the diagnosis of tendinitis. Sometimes X-rays are needed to rule out a bone injury. Treatment includes several days of rest and splinting of the affected area. Ice can be applied to reduce discomfort and swelling right after injury, and pain can be relieved with nonsteroidal anti-inflammatory drugs. After a few days of rest, gentle exercises can be done to increase the range of motion and flexibility of the joint. Often heat works better than ice at this point. Ultrasound or massage therapy may be recommended by your doctor. A recurrence can be avoided by warming up before exercise and cooling down afterward. In severe cases, an injection of corticosteroids may be recommended.

Trauma

Many problems in the musculoskeletal system are caused by injuries. They can result from sports activities or accidents and can affect most of the bones and joints in the body, although some are more susceptible than others. Examples of such injuries are fractures, sprains, and dislocations.

Fractures

A break in a bone is called a fracture. The break occurs as a result of the bone being stressed by physical forces greater than it can withstand. In a young person, the fracture usually occurs with a major injury, such as a motor vehicle accident or a sports-related injury. In older adults, fractures commonly occur with a fall. Adult bone gets weaker with age and will break with less force. Older women may suffer compression fractures of the vertebrae or fractures of the hip as a result of osteoporosis.

There are different types of fractures, classified according to the way the bone is broken:

- **Simple fractures** occur when the bone snaps but does not break the skin. (See Fig. 3.12A)
- **Open fractures** occur when the bone snaps and breaks through the skin. (See Fig. 3.12B)
- **Incomplete fractures** occur when the bone is cracked but not broken.

With all fractures, the first symptom is intense pain and swelling. A bruise may appear over a bone, and there may be numbness in the area. Pain becomes more severe when the affected area is moved or when pressure is applied. Fractures are diagnosed by physical examination and by X-ray. First aid involves giving support to the injured area and keeping it from moving with a splint. There is a risk of bone infection with an open fracture, so precautions should be taken to keep the injured area clean and to get prompt medical attention.

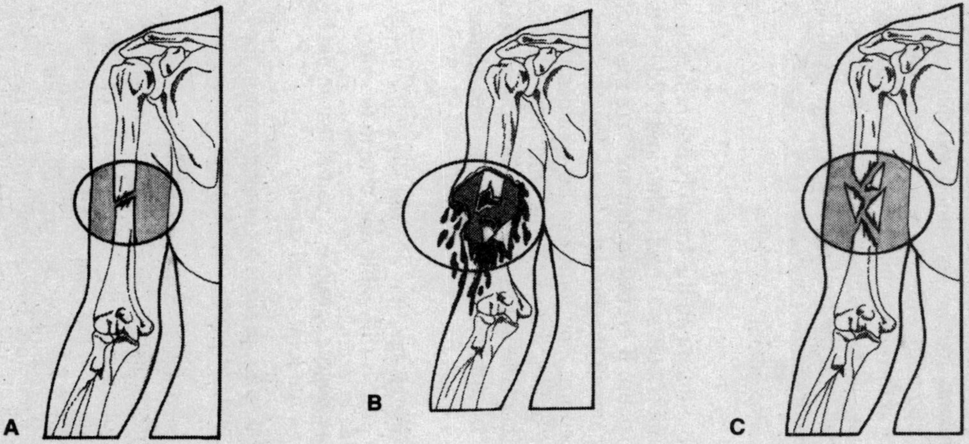

Figure 3.12 Fractures
Types of bone fractures include *simple* (or closed), in which the bone breaks in one place and the skin remains intact (left); *compound* (or open), in which the skin is broken and there is an open wound down to the level of the bone itself (middle); and *comminuted*, in which the bone breaks into several pieces (right).

Fractures are treated with a process called reduction, in which the ends of the bones are aligned. They can be manipulated back together by a physician's hands, or surgery can be performed and the bone ends can be secured with wires, pins, and metal plates. The broken bone is then immobilized by a cast or traction to allow healing. It takes about 6–8 weeks for a broken bone to mend, and the healing time is longer with large bones and with elderly patients.

Sprains

An injury to a ligament, the tough bands of fibrous tissue that connect bones to each other and hold joints in place, is a sprain. If excessive demands are made on a joint, the ligaments that hold the bones together may be stretched or torn. Any joint can be sprained, but the joints at the ankles, knees, wrists, and fingers are particularly susceptible to this type of injury. There are various types of sprains, depending on the degree of injury:

- **A first-degree sprain** is a minor stretching injury, but the joint is still stable and able to function.
- **A second-degree sprain** is a partial tear in the ligament, but the joint is still stable.
- **A third-degree sprain** is a complete tear in the ligament, and the joint is no longer stable.

Symptoms include pain and tenderness, swelling, and sometimes bruising. The amount of pain depends on the amount of injury. If the pain is severe or if weight cannot be borne on the joint, medical attention should be sought. An X-ray may be required to distinguish a sprain from a fracture. These problems are best treated with a basic approach known as RICE:

Rest;
Immobilization, such as using a splint;
Cold to reduce pain and swelling; and,
Elevation.

If pain is severe, if it persists, or if there are other symptoms present, immediate medical attention is required. A mild sprain can be supported with an elastic bandage on the joint. A second- or third-degree sprain may require a cast.

Dislocations

When two bones that make up a joint are no longer in contact, it is called a dislocation. This usually results from a major force great enough to tear the ligaments that support the joint. It can cause damage to the soft tissues that normally hold the joint in place. The main symptom is intense pain. The joint may look misshapen and become swollen, bruised, and immovable. Any joint can become dislocated, but this injury is most common in the shoulder, knee, hip, and fingers.

X-rays are done to show whether the bones are out of their normal position. The bones are repositioned in their normal place, possibly with the aid of an anesthetic to reduce pain. Sometimes surgery may be needed to reposition the bones and to repair damaged structures. Afterward, the joint will be immobilized for two or three weeks so the damaged tissues can heal. Sometimes dislocations can recur. It may be possible for the bones to be repositioned by the patient. This should be done under the guidance of a physician and evaluated afterward to ensure it was done properly.

Tumors

As with any cells of the body, bone cells are constantly reproducing so new cells can replace old ones. As with other parts of the body, bone cells can multiply and divide more than normal and result in tumors. These tumors may be benign (not cancerous) or cancerous, and they may arise in the bone or spread there from another source.

Benign Tumors

A benign tumor is one that stays localized to its original site and does not spread throughout the body.

Malignant Tumors

Malignant tumors invade and infiltrate local healthy tissue and damage or destroy that tissue. A primary malignancy refers to a tumor whose cells arise from the local area. Cancer cells that spread from another site are called metastatic or secondary tumors. Malignant tumors that begin in the bone are rare in adults. Secondary cancers in adults are most commonly from breast, kidney, lung, and thyroid cancer.

Soft tissue tumors are often first discovered as a lump or mass, while bone tumors frequently are discovered because a woman complains of a deep "boring" pain that interferes with sleep or activity. About 10 percent of bone cancer patients have fractures due to the weakening of bones by cancer cells. Diagnosis is based on a careful history, physical examination, and imaging studies, which may include X-ray, bone scans, CT, or MRI. A biopsy may be done so the cells can be examined under a microscope. The biopsy is usually performed by an orthopedic surgeon who specializes in oncology (tumors).

Treatment varies depending on whether the lesion is primary or metastatic. For a primary cancer, treatment often involves removing the cancer to prevent its spread. This can be done by a combination of surgery, radiation, and chemotherapy. Sometimes, artificial bone can be put in place of the bone that is removed. One of the major advances in the management of primary bone cancer has been the development of limb salvage techniques (See box).

Treatment of bone cancers that have arisen from cancer in other parts of the body is mostly geared to relieving pain, supporting the structure of the diseased bone, and maintaining the function of the limb. Depending on the type of cancer, it may first be treated with chemotherapy or hormonal agents. If there is a risk of fracture or if fracture has occurred, the bone may be repaired with metal implants.

LIMB SALVAGE

Amputation was the standard treatment for primary bone cancer for many years. Today new techniques in limb salvage have allowed many limbs to be saved. In this technique, the patient often receives chemotherapy to first shrink the tumor. The tumor is then removed along with some normal tissue to be sure no cancer cells are left behind. This leaves a large gap in the bone, which can be filled by a bone from a human body, by shortening of the limb, or by replacement with a custom-made metal joint. The type of reconstruction takes into consideration a number of factors, including the patient's needs, age, and lifestyle. Long-term studies have shown that this technique is as safe as amputation in most cases. It adds to the quality of a woman's life because her limb is spared and thus function is maintained.

Wrist Problems

The wrist is susceptible to damage from repetitive tasks, overuse, and injuries. Some of these problems are work-related and are thus hard to prevent. All wrist problems should receive prompt medical attention, however, so further injury can be prevented.

Carpal Tunnel Syndrome

This condition is caused by compression of the median nerve at the wrist, usually because of overuse. Extra fluid in the tissues around the joints and bone narrow the space between the joints and joint capsule, causing pressure. The condition is fairly common in women, especially those who are pregnant or are of middle age or older. It may occur in women with diabetes, thyroid disease, or rheumatoid arthritis. Workers who engage in repetitive tasks that involve movement of the wrist, strong grip, or exposure to vibration (typists, for instance) are especially at risk. Symptoms include hand and wrist pain, tingling, and thumb weakness. Numbness may occur in the thumb, and index, middle, and part of the ring fingers. Many women find the symptoms are worse at night. They may have a burning sensation that improves with shaking the hand. Many women note difficulty holding objects.

The history is critical to the diagnosis. Tests such as electromyography may be done to reproduce the symptoms and to measure responses of the muscles and nerves. Treatment is directed to treating any underlying medical problem, if present. Efforts should be made to eliminate any stress that may come from repetitive use. A splint may be used on the wrist, particularly at night. Medications such as NSAIDs and steroid injections may provide relief. In severe cases, a surgical procedure to release the constricting tunnel of fibers through which the nerve passes may be required.

DeQuervain's Tenosynovitis

This condition is an inflammation of the tendon sheaths that contain the muscles that lift the thumb. It is often seen in the last three months of pregnancy and immediately after pregnancy. Usually the patient has a history of chronic, repetitive movements of the wrist and thumb. Women often complain of a "triggering" sensation when they move their thumb. The diagnosis is based on the history and examination. Treatment involves keeping the thumb immobile with splints, nonsteroidal anti-inflammatory drugs, and occasionally injections of steroids. In severe cases, surgery may be required to release the tendon sheath.

TESTS AND PROCEDURES

Tests and procedures used to diagnose and treat the musculoskeletal system include imaging tests, tests to measure the responses of nerves and muscles, and surgical procedures. Imaging studies such as X-ray, CT scans, and MRI scans are often used, as well as specialized tests to study bone.

Bone Scans

This test uses radioisotopes to create images of areas inside the body. A small amount of radioactive material is injected into the bloodstream and gathers in specific parts of the body, depending on the element used. The element then breaks down in the body and produces gamma rays. These rays are reflected back into a special camera that creates an image of the area. Because gamma rays have good penetration through hard surfaces, they are useful in the study of bone. This test is often used to look for problems such as occult fractures, bone infection, and cancer.

Electromyography

This test is used to record the electrical properties of skeletal muscle. Electrodes are placed on the skin to measure whether the muscle is contracting. A small needle may be placed into muscle to assess normal or abnormal muscle responses while a muscle is at rest and while it is contracting. The results are shown on a video screen and audible signals are given to show the nature and location of any problem in the muscle. The response of the muscle also can be measured by electrical stimulation of the nerve to the muscle.

Arthroscopic Surgery

Fiberoptic technology has led to the development of the arthroscope, an instrument that allows a physician to look directly into a joint, diagnose problems, and often repair or relieve many of these problems at the same time.

The arthroscope is a long, thin metal tube that contains coated glass fibers and a series of magnifying lenses. The fibers carry light into the joint and relay a magnified image back to the operator. After anesthetic is administered (either local or general), a small cut is made into the joint. The arthroscope is then inserted through the incision, allowing the physician to view the joint either through an eye piece or on a video monitor. Once inside the joint a biopsy specimen also can be obtained and surgery performed.

Prior to arthroscopic surgery, surgeons opened joints to inspect and repair them. The joints were opened through long incisions, and wound healing and recovery of function required a great deal of time. Unlike traditional procedures, arthroscopy rarely takes more than an hour, and the patient can usually return home the same day. Most normal activities can be resumed in a week.

Joint Replacement Surgery

In a healthy joint, smooth, glistening cartilage covers the ends of bones and allows the bone ends to move smoothly and painlessly through a wide arc of motion. However, osteoarthritis, characterized by the breakdown of joint cartilage, occurs in many joints, particularly with aging. Although this can involve many joints, the hip, knee, and shoulder are usually affected.

Joint replacement surgery allows the surgeon to remove the diseased joint and replace it with a synthetic one. Like a healthy joint, the artificial one also has smooth gliding surfaces that allow painless joint motion.

Most joint replacements require replacement of both sides of the joint. For example, both the ball and the socket of the hip joint are often replaced in surgery for osteoarthritis. Sometimes after fracture only the ball portion of this ball and socket joint will be replaced. The decision of when to replace a diseased joint is based on a number of factors, including the degree of disability, lifestyle, age, and the patient's ability to withstand the risks of surgery.

Medications

Nonsteroidal anti-inflammatory drugs, NSAIDs, and corticosteroids are often used in treating disorders that cause swelling of joints and pain. In most cases, they relieve the pain but do not cure the problems. These drugs can bring relief, but they do have side effects and should be used with caution, especially long-term.

- NSAIDs include drugs such as aspirin, ibuprofen, and naproxen sodium that can be obtained without a prescription and are taken by mouth. They relieve pain and reduce inflammation. These drugs also may cause stomach upset or internal bleeding, so they should not be used by anyone who is anemic or has ulcers or kidney problems. Long-term use should be avoided.
- Corticosteroids are synthetic versions of hormones made in the adrenal gland that must be used under a doctor's direction. They reduce swelling, pain, redness, and heat. They can be taken by mouth, applied to the skin, dropped into the eye, or injected into an affected area. There is a risk of side effects with the long-term use of corticosteroids. These include weight gain, bone loss, muscle weakness, water retention, hypertension, and skin changes. Long-term use should not be stopped suddenly but rather slowly tapered off so the body can readjust.

PART IV

Cancer in Women

Claudia R. Baquet, M.D., M.P.H.

Cancer is characterized by an uncontrolled growth and spread of abnormal cells in the body. If not caught early, this proliferation of abnormal cells—called a tumor—can result in death. You should be aware, however, that cancer is not a hopeless disease, but one that can often be cured with prompt treatment. Recent advances in cancer therapy have led to nearly 50% of cancer patients remaining alive and free of disease some 5 years after the initial diagnosis.

Cancer occurs in larger numbers among the elderly. It is much more common in people over 65; about 73 million Americans are eventually expected to develop cancer in their later lives. Lung cancer is the leading cause of cancer-related deaths in both men and women, followed by breast cancer in women. The incidence rates and the death rates vary in men and women and in different ethnic groups, based on the type of cancer.

CAUSES OF CANCER

Why does cancer occur? What triggers an occurrence? The reasons are still largely unknown, although the mechanisms of the disease have long been recognized.

The body renews and replaces its cells through a constant process of cell division and growth. Cells exist, repair themselves, die, and are reborn. Old tissues are replaced with new, injuries are repaired, and the body grows and develops. Normally, the body has control mechanisms that limit abnormal cell growth. Cancer cells, however, continue to grow without restraint, dividing many more times than do normal cells. The abnormal cells form tumors, which compete with normal, healthy tissue for nutrients.

Tumors can be benign (harmless) or malignant.

Benign tumors can be removed with surgery and usually do not recur. Malignant tumors, on the other hand, can grow, invade, and destroy nearby areas of the body. They can spread, or metastasize, to distant organs and form new tumors. If malignant tumors aren't removed or killed early in their development, they can spread to other parts of the body.

Some cancers spread quickly, whereas others develop slowly. Because cancers can be most successfully treated before they spread, it is important to be aware of cancer warning signs and steps that can be taken for early detection of the disease.

METHODS OF EARLY DETECTION

The American Cancer Society has identified certain warning signs that should alert you to see your doctor promptly (see "The Seven Warning Signs of Cancer"). None of these signs necessarily means that you have cancer, but each one is important and warrants immediate medical attention. Pain is seldom a symptom of early types of cancer, so don't wait until it hurts if the other symptoms don't disappear on their own.

Certain tests can also help detect cancer in early stages. These screening tests are often done routinely for people who may have symptoms of a disease and for those who have risk factors, such as age and family history. Every woman should have a physical examination annually and undergo the following routine screening tests as needed.

- Pelvic exam and Pap test (annually after age 18 or once sexual activity has begun) to detect cancer of the cervix, ovary, or uterus.
- Mammography (every 1–2 years from age 40 to

49; yearly thereafter) to detect cancer of the breast. High-risk women may benefit from earlier screening

- Fecal occult blood test (annually after age 50) to detect hidden blood in the stool, which may be a sign of cancer of the colon and rectum
- Sigmoidoscopy (every 3 to 5 years after age 50) to detect changes in the colon or rectum that could be a sign of colon and rectal cancer

These tests may be done earlier in women who have special risks. For instance, if you have a family history of cancer of the breast or colon, you will benefit from having tests to detect these diseases more than women who have no family history of disease. Colonoscopy, a test used to view the inside of the entire colon, is recommended in women age 40 and older who have had inflammatory bowel disease or who have a family member who had cancer of the colon or rectum at an early age.

Be alert to any changes in your body. Besides scheduling a yearly pelvic exam, you should regularly examine your breasts. Many breast lumps have been found through self-examination. It is best to do the breast examination at the same point in your menstrual cycle each month (or on the same day of the month if you're postmenopausal), because breast tissue changes with your cycle. It will be easier for you to detect anything unusual if you follow this suggestion. Check out other areas of your body, including your skin, for any suspicious signs.

Have your mouth checked periodically by a dentist. In addition, use a mirror to examine your mouth. Changes in the color of the gums, lips, or cheeks as well as sores, swelling, bleeding, or thickening of any tissue should be reviewed by your doctor.

RISK FACTORS OF CANCER

About 80 percent of all cancers may be related to the things we eat, drink, and smoke and to the quality of our environment and workplace. Repeated and long-term contact with cancer-causing agents (carcinogens) can damage cells or change cells that are already damaged and lead to cancer. For example, tobacco smoke is one of the most potent carcinogens, and it acts with other elements, such as alcohol, to increase the risk of certain cancers.

Tobacco

Smoking is a major risk factor for cancer. The risk of dying from lung cancer is 12 times greater in a smoker than in a nonsmoker. Overall, smoking causes 30 percent of all deaths from cancer. In addition to contributing to lung cancer, it also increases the risk of cancers of the cervix, mouth, throat, esophagus, pancreas, bladder,

THE SEVEN WARNING SIGNS OF CANCER

1. Change in bowel or bladder habits
2. A sore that does not heal
3. Unusual bleeding or discharge
4. Thickening or lump in the breast or elsewhere
5. Indigestion or difficulty swallowing
6. Obvious change in a wart or mole
7. Nagging cough or hoarseness

and possibly the stomach. Smokers also have a higher rate of cardiovascular and respiratory disease. Those who live with smokers are also at risk for cancer.

If you smoke, quit. As soon as you stop smoking, your risk of cancer decreases.

Diet

A high-fat diet has been linked to certain types of cancer, including cancer of the breast, colon, rectum, and ovaries. Obesity has been linked to increased cancer death rates. The exact link between diet and cancer is not clear, but most health practitioners agree that it is best to eat a variety of foods, to limit saturated fats and cholesterol, and to eat foods high in fiber. Eating fresh fruits and vegetables daily may decrease your risk of cancer by as much as 50 percent. An increased daily intake of vitamins A, C, and E may also boost your protection against lung cancer.

Sunlight

One of the most common forms of cancer in the United States is skin cancer, which is caused by exposure to ultraviolet (UV) radiation from the sun. Repeated exposure to the sun may be especially harmful for people who have fair skin or who burn or freckle easily. Take steps now to avoid the sun, especially between the hours of 10:00 A.M. and 2:00 P.M., when the sun's rays are strongest. If you are out at that time, wear protective clothing, including a hat. Use sunscreen to block the UV light. Remember, a tan is really the body's attempt to protect itself against the sun.

Alcohol

Cancers of the mouth, throat, esophagus, and liver occur more often among heavy drinkers, especially those who smoke as well. Alcohol also poses a number of other health problems. If you regularly drink more than two drinks a day, you should probably consider cutting back or stopping drinking altogether.

Chemicals

Exposure to certain industrial agents or chemicals increases the risk of various types of cancer. Exposure to these chemicals may occur in the workplace, outdoors, or at home. They include

- Asbestos fibers
- Nickel, chromate, and vinylchloride
- Solvent cleaners, cleaning fluids, and paint thinners
- Lawn and garden chemicals (pesticides and fungicides)

Avoid inhaling any of these chemicals, especially in areas that are not well ventilated. Read labels carefully and avoid having these agents come in contact with your skin or household items.

Hormones

Certain cancers are stimulated by an excess of the female hormone estrogen. Estrogen occurs naturally in reproductive-age women. It is also the main component of birth control pills and hormone-replacement therapy after menopause. Birth control pills have not been linked to cancer in most women, however, and they may even protect against some types of cancer. Replacement of estrogen alone can increase the risk of endometrial cancer in postmenopausal women, but when it is combined with the hormone progesterone, the risk is lowered. Before taking estrogen, discuss the risks with your physician.

Genetics

Some cancers may be inherited. The risk of breast, colon, and skin cancer, for instance, is higher in some families than in others. Your risk for these cancers is high if you have a first-degree relative (mother, father, sister or brother) who developed one of these cancers. If you have close relatives who have had cancer, tell your doctor. He or she may advise that you receive regular checkups and tests.

TYPES OF CANCER

Cancer in women can be nongynecologic or gynecologic. *Nongynecologic* cancers occur in both men and women. *Gynecologic* cancers, however, are unique to women; they occur in the female reproductive and genital organs. (Although breast cancer can occur in both men and women, it is considered here as a gynecologic cancer, because it is much more common in women than in men.) For more details about all of these cancers, see the sections where the specific body parts are discussed. (See Fig. 4.1).

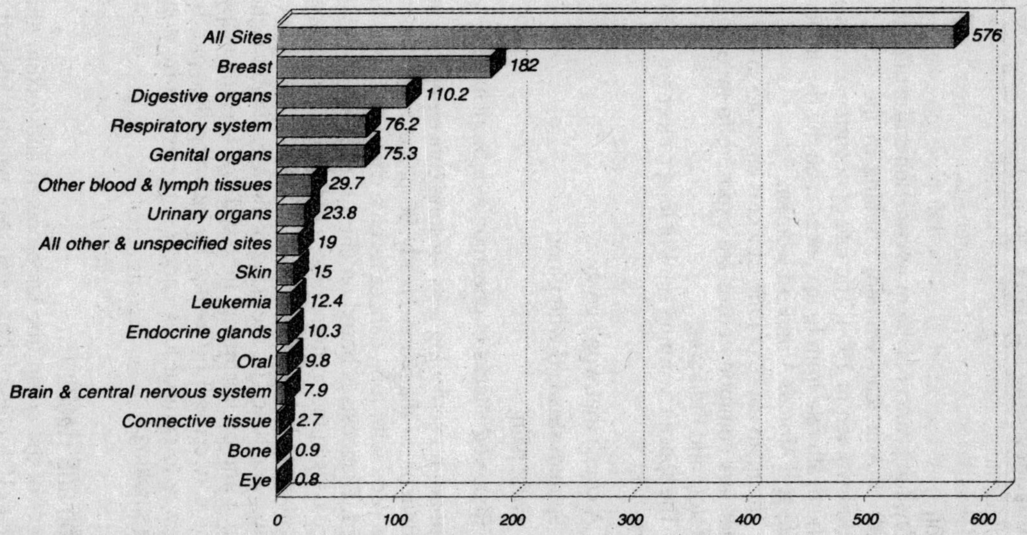

Figure 4.1 Estimated New Cancer Cases and Deaths in Women, 1994.

Nongynecologic Cancers

Lung

Today, lung cancer is the most common cause of cancer death in American women, resulting in the death of 59,000 women in 1994. The rate of occurrence as well as the death rate from lung cancer is on the rise in both white and African-American women.

The main cause of lung cancer is cigarette smoking. Other less common causes are exposure to radon gas, asbestos, and radiation.

The specific warning signs of lung cancer are as follows:

- A cough that won't go away
- Sputum streaked with blood
- Chest pain
- Repeated attacks of pneumonia or bronchitis

There are no screening tests for lung cancer, and it can be difficult to diagnose. Nearly 90 percent of patients diagnosed with lung cancer receive care too late to be cured. Diagnosis is based on chest X-rays, examination of the cells in the sputum, biopsy of the suspicious area, and imaging tests of the bronchial tubes. Survival rates are low and based on the stage of disease. Surgery is the main form of treatment, followed by chemotherapy. Some cancers will be treated by radiation therapy. The best way to combat lung cancer is prevention by stopping smoking.

Colon and Rectum

Cancer of the colon (the large bowel) and rectum (the last 8 to 10 inches of the large bowel, which leads to the anus) is the second most common cancer in women.

Although the death rate from colon and rectum cancer is decreasing in white women, it is remaining steady for African-American women. This form of cancer occurs more often in older women, in those who have a history of inflammatory bowel disease, and in women who have a family history of cancer of the colon or rectum. A diet high in saturated fat and low in fiber appears to increase the risk of this disease, and increased daily intake of fiber, fruits, and vegetables seems to protect against it.

Cancer of the colon and rectum can be detected early. The following persistent symptoms are warning signs of a possible problem:

- Diarrhea or constipation (recurring or alternating)
- Blood in or on the stool
- Stools that are narrower than usual, indicating obstruction
- General abdominal discomfort (bloating, fullness, or cramps)
- Frequent gas pains
- A feeling that the bowel doesn't empty completely

These symptoms could be a sign of a number of things, so it's important to ascertain the cause without delay. The diagnosis is based on a physical examination and tests that detect blood in the stool or growths in the colon or rectum. Sometimes a piece of a growth can be removed for further study (biopsy). The most common treatment for bowel cancer includes surgical removal of the diseased area, and follow-up chemotherapy may be recommended.

Bladder

Each year, more than 13,000 American women will be diagnosed with bladder cancer. If the disease is treated early, the cure rate is good. Cancer of the bladder is twice as likely to occur in women who smoke as in women who don't smoke. The main symptom is blood in the urine and the need to urinate more often than normal. Pain rarely occurs in the early stages, and there may be no symptoms at all.

Diagnosis is based on physical examination, laboratory tests, and imaging studies. A urine sample may reveal cancer cells. Since the cancer usually occurs inside the bladder, a test may be done using a thin lighted tube that is inserted inside the bladder. A sample of any growth may be removed for further study. Bladder cancer is usually treated surgically.

Skin

Skin cancer is the most common form of cancer in the United States, with about 700,000 new cases annually. It is estimated that 40 to 50 percent of Americans who live to age 65 will have skin cancer at least once. Caused by exposure to ultraviolet light, skin cancer occurs more often in regions that traditionally have more sunlight. Basal cell carcinoma, a slow-growing cancer that usually does not spread to other parts of the body, accounts for more than 90 percent of all skin cancers. It usually appears as pale bumps or red scaly patches. Squamous cell skin cancer can spread to other areas and must be removed surgically. Multiple melanoma is invasive and life threatening. It first appears as a molelike growth that gets bigger, darker, and more inflamed. (See Fig. 4.2)

Warning signs of skin cancer include

- A change in the size or color of a mole or wart
- Scaliness, oozing, or bleeding
- Itchiness, tenderness, or pain in a bump or a mole
- A sore that does not heal

Regular self-examination is the best way to detect skin cancers. Inspect all moles carefully and look for any changes. Examine all parts of the body, because melanoma can appear in places that have not been exposed to sunlight. The cure rate is nearly 100 percent if skin cancers are treated before they spread.

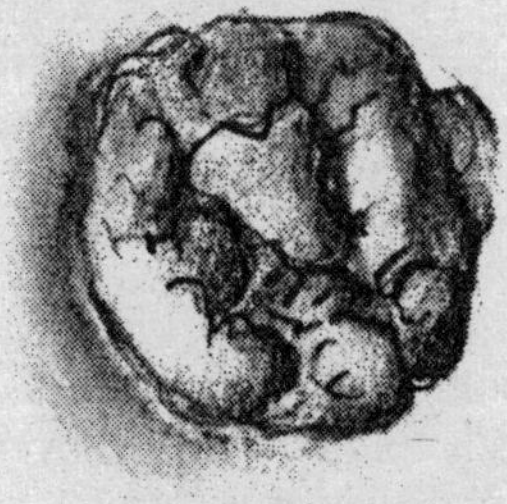

Figure 4.2 Skin Cancer.
Basal cell cancer is the most common type of cancer and looks like pale bumps or red patches.

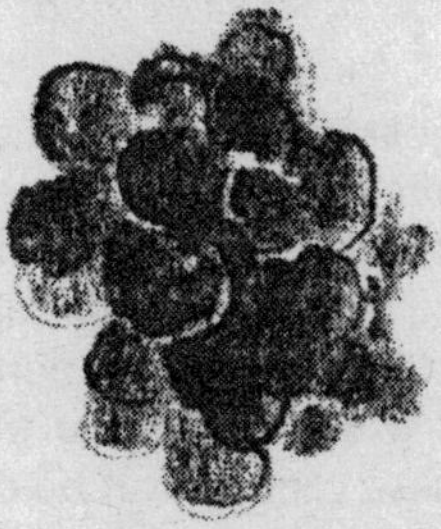

Melanoma is a less common but more severe type of skin cancer that looks like a mole but grows bigger and darker.

Pancreas

The pancreas, a large gland located behind the stomach and in front of the spine, makes enzymes that digest food as well as insulin, which controls the amount of sugar in the blood.

Cancer of the pancreas is a common cause of death in women. It is known as a *silent* disease, because there are no symptoms in the early stages. As a result, the cancer has often spread by the time it is diagnosed, which makes for low survival rates. Symptoms are pain in the upper abdomen and sometimes the back, nausea, loss of appetite, weight loss, and weakness.

Oral

Cancers of the mouth, lips, gums, cheeks, teeth, jaw, and tongue are usually found in people over age 45. The best way to detect oral cancer is through self-examination. Look for the following warning signs:

- A sore that bleeds easily and doesn't heal
- A lump or thickening
- A red or white patch that doesn't go away
- Difficulty chewing, swallowing, or moving tongue or jaws

Women who smoke, especially if they also drink alcohol, are at an increased risk for oral cancer.

Diagnosis is established by taking a biopsy of any lump or abnormal area and examining it under a microscope. Imaging tests also may be done to see if the disease has spread to other parts of the body. If caught early, many of these cancers can be cured.

Gynecologic Cancers

Breast

Breast cancer is occurring in epidemic proportions in the United States. About one of every nine women will develop breast cancer during her lifetime. African-American women, who are less likely than white women to develop breast cancer, are more likely than white women to die from it. Formerly, it had been thought that African-American women postponed seeing a doctor or did not have access to care, resulting in the disease being diagnosed in later stages. Recent research, however, indicates that a more aggressive form of the disease may afflict African-American women, particularly younger ones.

Women who have a mother or a sister who has had breast cancer are at increased risk of getting the disease. The risk is also higher in women who have not had children or who had children later in life. Breast cancer has also been linked with alcohol use and a high-fat diet.

The best way to detect breast cancer is by doing a monthly self-examination, seeing a doctor annually for an examination, and by having periodic mammograms. The warning signs of breast cancer are

- Changes in the breast that don't disappear—a lump, thickening, swelling, or dimpling
- Irritation of breast skin
- Nipple distortion, retraction, or scaliness
- Discharge from the nipple

The earlier breast cancer can be found and treated, the better the chance of cure. Breast cancer can spread to the bones, liver, lungs, or brain, making it very difficult to treat in later stages.

The first stage in diagnosis is feeling for any breast lumps. Your doctor may use a needle to withdraw fluid or a piece of the lump so that it can be studied in a laboratory. Treatment of breast cancer depends on how advanced the cancer is at the time of diagnosis.

Cervix

The cervix, the narrow neck of a woman's uterus, can go through a series of changes that eventually can lead to cancer. Cervical cancer is the third most common form of cancer of the female genital tract and accounts for 19 percent of these cancers. Cervical cancer occurs almost twice as often in younger African-American than in age-matched white women; over the age of 65, African-American women develop cervical cancer about three times more often than white women. Death rates follow similar patterns, with African-American women dying more often from the disease.

Risk factors for cancer of the cervix include having sex at an early age, having multiple sexual partners, and smoking. Women without any of these risk factors can also develop cervical cancer, however.

A precancerous or localized condition of the cervix can develop over time into invasive cancer. There may be no warning signs with early cervical cancer. More advanced cervical cancer can be signaled by abnormal bleeding or vaginal discharge. Changes in the cervix can be detected through regular Pap tests. Precancerous changes in the cervix can be treated before they become cancerous.

To confirm the diagnosis, a biopsy is done. A sample of tissue from the cervix is removed and studied under a microscope. If detected early, the cancer can be removed surgically. For prevention, always have a Pap smear test done at least once a year after the age of 18.

Endometrium (Uterus)

Cancer of the uterus accounts for 5 percent of all cancers in women and is the most common gynecologic cancer. Most cancers of the uterus occur in the endometrium, the lining of the uterus.

Endometrial cancer occurs most often in older women; it is rare before age 40. Cancer of the endometrium is more likely to affect women who are infertile, began menstruating at an early age, don't have children, have menstrual problems, and go through menopause at a later age. Other risk factors include obesity, diabetes mellitus, hypertension, and use of estrogen. Gallbladder disease and thyroid disease may also be associated with increased risk.

The most common symptom of cancer of the endometrium is abnormal bleeding or discharge from the vagina. Because this disease often occurs in women around the age of menopause, they may mistake this symptom for a menstrual period. Any bleeding or discharge that appears after menopause should be checked by a doctor.

Cancer of the endometrium is diagnosed by removing a piece of the lining of the uterus for further study. A hysterectomy (removal of the uterus) is the usual treatment.

Ovary

The ovaries are located on either side of the uterus; each month during ovulation one of the ovaries releases an egg. These glands also produce estrogen. Cancer of the ovary is the second most common gynecologic cancer and the fourth leading cause of death from cancer among women.

Risk factors for cancer of the ovary include a family history of the disease. It generally develops after menopause and is seen more often in women who have had no children or who had trouble conceiving. It is often hard to detect until it is in the advanced stages, when the following warning signs occur.

- Discomfort in the pelvic region
- Indigestion, gas, or bloating
- Pain during intercourse
- Abnormal vaginal bleeding
- Pain and swelling in the abdomen

There is no good method of screening for cancer of the ovary, although the use of two tests, ultrasound and a blood test for a protein called CA125, show promise. Any abnormality should be checked by a doctor. Imaging tests may be done to get a better idea of the size of a growth. Surgery to remove the ovary, and any other affected organs, is an important part of treatment.

Vulva and Vagina

Cancer of the vulva and vagina are rare and occur most often in older women. Warning signs include a lump or sore on the vulva (external genitals) or in the vagina.

Risk of vaginal cancer is increased after radiation of the cervix, chronic irritation, and uterine exposure to the hormone DES. Diagnosis is determined by removing a sample of tissue for further study. If detected in the early stages, cancers of the vulva and the vagina can be treated successfully.

TYPES OF CANCER TREATMENT

Although a diagnosis of cancer is serious, it no longer carries the dire consequences it once did. Nearly 50% of all patients diagnosed with cancer can now be cured because of advances in early detection and treatment.

The type of treatment is based on the stage of disease. It can involve surgery, radiation therapy, chemotherapy, or a combination of these. Emotional support is invaluable in helping patients with cancer deal with the physical and psychological aspects of their disease.

At the time of diagnosis, the extent of the disease is determined. Called *staging,* this is a useful way to determine whether cancer is localized or has spread to other areas. Additional staging is used to determine types of treatment and possible outcomes. One method of classification is *historical stage,* which relates the extent of cancer at the time of diagnosis to the natural history of the disease. The *localized stage* refers to a cancer that is confined to its place of origin. The *regional stage* refers to disease that has spread beyond its place of origin to surrounding areas. The *distant stage* is cancer that has spread extensively to distant tissues or organs.

For localized cancer, surgery is often used to remove the affected tissues. During the surgery, a lymph node or nodes may be removed for examination to see if cancer has spread to the lymphatic system, where it can be spread to other parts of the body.

Radiation therapy is another form of local therapy. Treatment can be directed to particular areas of the body, or radioactive units can be implanted at the site of the cancer. For other cancers, the whole body may receive radiotherapy. Radiation can be used occasionally before surgery to shrink tumors or after surgery to destroy any remaining cancer cells.

Drug therapy, known as chemotherapy, uses drugs to destroy cancer cells. These chemicals interfere with the cells' ability to grow and multiply. The drugs may be administered orally or intravenously. Chemotherapy can destroy healthy cells as well as cancer cells. Side effects of chemotherapy vary and are strongly related to the specific drug or drugs given as well as the type and extent of disease.

Antihormonals block the body's production of specific hormones. The growth of some cancers is stimulated by hormones, and antihormonal drugs limit that stimulation. One such drug is tamoxifen, which is used to treat some breast cancer. Because this drug interferes with the actions of estrogen, women who take it may develop symptoms of menopause.

Some types of cancer therapy have side effects, some more severe than others. Many side effects are temporary, and many can be successfully managed so that the patient is as comfortable as possible.

THE FUTURE OF CANCER RESEARCH AND CANCER CARE

Research in new areas of cancer prevention and treatment is ongoing. One area of research is directed toward examining cancer at the molecular level. By identifying genes that may cause cancer or may make one more susceptible to cancer, scientists hope to be able to target people who are at risk so they can receive early treatment and may even be able to avoid getting cancer at all.

Other research efforts are being directed toward antioxidants, chemicals that consume free radicals, which are waste products produced by our bodies. Some evidence suggests that free radicals may cause cell damage and degeneration. Other research is trying to find ways to boost the body's natural immune response, so it can fight cancer wherever it appears in the body.

THE AFTERMATH OF CANCER: WHAT YOU CAN DO

Cancer changes the life of the person who has it as well as the lives of the family and friends of that person. If you suffer from cancer, you may have initially reacted to the disease with anger and denial and now feel a range of emotions from hope to despair. More important, you may feel that you have suffered physical and emotional losses that you find hard to deal with and that prevent you from moving ahead to continue on with your life.

Support groups, psychologists and psychiatrists, and families and friends are important recovery resources.

EDITORS AND CONTRIBUTORS

MEDICAL CO-EDITORS

ROSELYN PAYNE EPPS, M.D., M.P.H., M.A., F.A.A.P., is an expert at the National Institutes of Health, Bethesda, Maryland, and a Professor at Howard University College of Medicine, Washington, D.C. She is recognized nationally and internationally in areas of health policy and research, health promotion and disease prevention, and medical education and health service delivery. As a pioneer and leader in numerous professional and community organizations, she served, in 1991, as the first African-American president of AMWA and the founding president of the AMWA Foundation.

SUSAN COBB STEWART, M.D., F.A.C.P., is an internist and gastroenterologist, and is presently Associate Medical Director at J. P. Morgan in New York, where she delivers general medical care, specialty consultations, and preventive services. She is Clinical Assistant Professor of Medicine at SUNY, Brooklyn. Since serving as President of AMWA in 1990, Dr. Stewart has continued to help AMWA shape and focus its mission in the area of women's health.

CONTRIBUTORS

Judith C. Ahronheim, M.D., F.A.C.P., a nationally recognized specialist in geriatrics, is Attending Physician at Mount Sinai Medical Center in New York. She is also Associate Professor of Medicine and Associate Professor of Geriatrics at Mount Sinai School of Medicine. Dr. Ahronheim serves on the Ethics Committee of the American Geriatrics Society.

Claudia R. Baquet, M.D., M.P.H., serves as Visiting Scholar in Health Policy and Assistant Dean for Health Affairs at the University of Maryland School of Medicine in Baltimore, Maryland. She developed and implemented the first national cancer prevention and control intervention research program that focuses solely on African-American and Native American populations.

Carolyn Barley Britton, M.D., M.S., is an Associate Professor of Clinical Neurology and an Associate Attending Physician at Columbia Presbyterian Medical Center. She is Director of Ambulatory Care for the Department of Neurology. She has served on the New York State Advisory Council to the AIDS Institute.

Judith J. Petry, M.D., F.A.C.S., is a former Assistant Professor of Plastic and Reconstructive Surgery at the University of Massachusetts Medical School. She has recently retired from the private practice of plastic surgery in Massachusetts and now resides in Vermont.

Francesca Morosani Thompson, M.D., F.A.A.O.S., is Associate Attending Surgeon at St. Luke's/Roosevlt Hospital Center and Chief of the Adult Orthopaedic Foot Clinic at Roosevelt Hospital in New York. She is also an Assistant Clinical Professor of Orthopaedic Surgery at the College of Physicians and Surgeons of Columbia University. Dr. Thompson is on the Board of Directors of the American Orthopaedic Foot and Ankle Society.

Laura L. Tosi, M.D., F.A.A.O.S., is an Assistant Professor of Pediatrics and Orthopaedic Surgery at the George Washington School of Medicine and the Children's National Medical Center in Washington, D.C. She was the second woman to be elected to the Board of Directors of the American Academy of Orthopaedic Surgeons. She is also a past president of the Ruth Jackson Orthopaedic Society.

Patience White, M.D., F.A.A.P., is Director of the Adult and Pediatric Rheumatology Division at George Washington University Hospital and Children's National Medical Center, Washington, D.C. She is a Professor of Medicine and Pediatrics at George Washington University Medical School.

INDEX